THE ULTIMATE KETOGENIC COOKBOOK

BEST COOKIES RECIPES FOR YOUR VEGAN DIET THAT HELP YOU TO LOSE WEIGHT AND KEEP YOU HEALTHY.

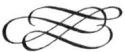

MELISSA WALTRIP

COPYRIGHT

© Copyright 2021 by Melissa Waltrip

All rights reserved.

This document is geared towards providing exact and reliable information concerning the topic and issue covered. The publication is sold with the idea that the publisher is not required to render accounting, officially permitted or otherwise qualified services. If advice is necessary, legal or professional, a practiced individual in the profession should be ordered.

- From a Declaration of Principles which was accepted and approved equally by a Committee of the American Bar Association and a Committee of Publishers and Associations.

In no way is it legal to reproduce, duplicate, or transmit any part of this document in either electronic means or printed format. Recording of this publication is strictly prohibited, and any storage of this document is not allowed unless with written permission from the publisher. All rights reserved.

The information provided herein is stated to be truthful and consistent, in that any liability, in terms of inattention or otherwise, by any usage or abuse of any policies, processes, or directions contained within is the solitary and utter responsibility of the recipient reader. Under no circumstances will any legal responsibility or blame be held against the publisher for any reparation, damages, or monetary loss due to the information herein, either directly or indirectly.

Respective authors own all copyrights not held by the publisher.

The information herein is offered for informational purposes solely and is universal as so. The presentation of the information is without a contract or any guarantee assurance.

The trademarks that are used are without any consent, and the publication of the trademark is without permission or backing by the trademark owner. All trademarks and brands within this book are for clarifying purposes only and are owned by the owners themselves, not affiliated with this document.

CONTENTS

VEGAN RECIPES

1. VEGAN PHO — 3
2. VEGGIE PILAF WITH VEGAN SAUSAGES — 6
3. VEGAN GINGERBREAD — 8
4. VEGAN CARBONARA — 10
5. VEGAN SCONES — 12
6. VEGAN GINGERBREAD DOUGHNUTS — 14
7. VEGAN ZUCCHINI FRITTERS — 16
8. VEGAN PESTO GNOCCHI — 18
9. VEGAN MUSHROOM BOURGUIGNON — 20
10. VEGAN BUFFALO WINGS — 22
11. VEGAN INDIAN CURRY — 24
12. VEGAN SPINACH AND FETTA PIE — 26
13. TARTE TATIN TOMATO VEGAN — 28
14. VEGAN CUPCAKES WITH CARAMEL POPCORN — 30
15. LEMON AND BLUEBERRY VEGAN TART — 32
16. VEGAN SPINACH FILO SCROLL — 34
17. VEGAN CHOCOLATE LAVA CAKES — 36
18. VEGAN MANGO JELLY SLICE — 38
19. VEGAN CHOC MOUSSE EGGS — 40
20. VEGAN LEMON TARTS — 42
21. VEGAN QUINOA PILAF — 45
22. VEGAN OREO CUPCAKES — 47
23. VEGAN BURGER IN A LETTUCE BUN — 49
24. VEGAN ROASTED CAULIFLOWER SALAD — 51
25. VEGAN CHOC-CHIP COOKIES — 53
26. ULTIMATE VEGAN BREAKFAST WRAP — 55
27. EASY VEGAN BOLOGNAISE — 57
28. LIME AND RASPBERRY VEGAN CHEESECAKE — 59
29. VEGAN PASTA NOURISH BOWL — 61
30. VEGAN PANCAKE RECIPE — 63

31. HEALTHY VEGAN TACOS	65
32. VEGAN VANILLA SLICE	67
33. LEMON AND LIME VEGAN TARTS	69
34. VEGAN CHOCOLATE	71
35. VEGAN MEDITERRANEAN	73
36. CRISPY VEGAN NOODLE SALAD	75
37. VEGAN CHICKPEA SATAY CURRY	77
38. VEGAN STUFFED ROAST PUMPKIN	79
39. VEGAN 'ICED VOVO' FROZEN CHEESECAKE	81
40. SATAY NOODLE STIR-FRY VEGAN	83
41. VEGAN 'MEATBALL' SKEWERS WITH GREEN HUMMUS	85
42. VEGAN AND GLUTEN-FREE CHRISTMAS CAKE	87
43. VEGAN JAPANESE STUFFED SWEET POTATOES	89
44. VEGAN SOBA NOODLE SALAD WITH SPICY PEANUT DRESSING	91
45. CREAMY VEGAN SUN-DRIED TOMATO AND BROCCOLINI GNOCCHI	93
46. CREAMY VEGAN TOMATO SOUP WITH SPINACH AND RICOTTA RAVIOLI	95
47. ICE-CUBE TRAY VEGAN CHEESECAKE BITES	97
48. PLANT POWER POTATO SALAD WITH VEGAN DRESSING	99
49. VEGAN TAHINI BISCUITS	101
50. VEGAN CHICKPEA SATAY CURRY	103
51. CREAMY VEGAN TOMATO SOUP WITH SPINACH AND RICOTTA RAVIOLI	105
52. CREAMY VEGAN SUN-DRIED TOMATO AND BROCCOLINI GNOCCHI	107
53. VEGAN STUFFED ROAST PUMPKIN	109

COOKIES RECIPES

1. CUTE CRITTER COOKIES	113
2. ALMOND AND CHERRY COOKIES	115
3. BANANA COOKIES	117
4. TRASH COOKIES	119
5. MILO THUMBPRINT COOKIES	121
6. APRICOT AND PISTACHIO COOKIES	123

7. CHOCOLATE AND COCONUT COOKIES	125
8. CHOCOLATE CHILLI COOKIES	127
9. EASY KITKAT COOKIES	129
10. CHOCKY ROCK COOKIES	131
11. CRANBERRY LEMON COOKIES	133
12. TAHINI AND HONEY COOKIES	135
13. CHOC DIPPED FORTUNE COOKIES	137
14. VEGAN CHOC-CHIP COOKIES	139
15. PEANUT BUTTER SANDWICH COOKIES	141
16. SUPER-EASY JELLY COOKIES	143
17. CRUNCHY NUTTY CORNFLAKE COOKIES	145
18. BAILEY'S CHOCOLATE CHIP COOKIES	147
19. SANTA PULL-APART COOKIES	149
20. ROCKY ROAD CAKE MIX COOKIES	152
21. PEAR AND WHITE CHOC MISO COOKIES	154
22. CHOCOLATE AND CANDY CANE CRUSH COOKIES	156
23. CRUNCHY CHOC-CHIP MICROWAVE COOKIES	158
24. DOUBLE CHOC-CHIP KALE COOKIES	160
25. MUESLI COOKIES	162
26. SNOWFLAKE COOKIES	164
27. CHOC-CHIP COOKIE MASH-UP	166
28. PEANUT AND CHOC CHIP COOKIE CAKE	168
29. COOKIES AND CREAM MIXED BERRY CRUMBLES	170
30. DATE AND CHOC-CHIP COOKIE BARS	172
31. SPICED GINGER COOKIES	174

VEGAN RECIPES

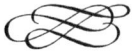

VEGAN PHO

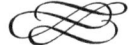

INGREDIENTS

- 200g dried flat rice noodles
- 2 x 200g pkts Thai marinated tofu
- 1 bunch choy sum, ends trimmed, cut into 4cm lengths
- 100g bean sprouts
- Mint leaves, to serve
- Coriander leaves, to serve
- PHO BROTH
- 4 shallots, peeled, halved
- 5cm-piece ginger, peeled, cut into quarters
- 1 cinnamon stick or quill
- 2 whole star anise
- 6 whole cloves
- 1 tsp black peppercorns
- 1 large carrot, peeled, halved
- 3/4 cup (20g) dried sliced shiitake mushrooms
- 4 cups (1L) Coles Vegan Chicken Style Stock
- 2 tbs soy sauce

METHOD

Step 1: To make the pho broth, place the shallot and ginger in a frying pan over medium-high heat. Cook, stirring occasionally, for 3 mins or until browned. Add cinnamon, star anise, cloves and peppercorns and cook, stirring, for 1 min or until aromatic. Transfer to a slow cooker. Add carrot, mushroom, stock and 4 cups (1L) water. Cover and cook for 4 hours on high (or 6 hours on low).

Step 2 :Use a slotted spoon to remove the shallot, ginger, cinnamon and star anise. Discard. Remove carrot. Slice and return to the slow cooker. Stir in the soy sauce.

Step 3 :Place noodles in a large heatproof bowl and cover with boiling water. Set aside for 5 mins to soak. Drain.

Step 4 :Add the tofu, noodles and choy sum to the slow cooker. Cover and cook for 10 mins or until heated through.

Step 5 :Divide the noodle mixture among serving bowls. Top with bean sprouts, mint and coriander.

RECIPE NOTES

(+ 5 mins soaking time).

SERVE WITH sliced spring onion, sriracha or chilli sauce and lime wedges

On the stove

To make this without a slow cooker, cook the broth, covered, in a saucepan over low heat for 1 hour, stirring occasionally. Add noodles, choy sum and tofu. Cook for 10 mins.

VEGGIE PILAF WITH VEGAN SAUSAGES

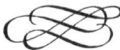

INGREDIENTS

- 2 tbs olive oil
- 1 large brown onion, thinly sliced
- 2 garlic cloves, crushed
- 1 tsp ground turmeric
- 2/3 cup (145g) brown basmati rice
- 2 cups (500ml) vegetable stock
- 400g can lentils, rinsed, drained
- 1/4 cup (35g) currants
- 300g pkt Coles Australian Superfood Stir-Fry
- 300g pkt kale and cashew vegan sausages
- Coriander sprigs, to serve
- Coconut yoghurt, to serve

METHOD

Step 1 :Heat the oil in a large non-stick frying pan over medium-high heat. Add onion and cook, stirring, for 3-4 mins or until onion softens. Add garlic and turmeric and cook for 30 secs or until aromatic. Add the rice and stir to combine.

Step 2 :Add stock, lentils and currants to the onion mixture in the pan and bring to a simmer. Reduce heat to medium-low. Cover and cook for 15 mins or until rice is tender. Add the stir-fry vegetables and use a fork to gently toss until the vegetables are just tender. Cover and set aside for 2-3 mins to steam. Season.

Step 3 :Meanwhile, spray a separate large non-stick frying pan with olive oil spray. Cook the sausages following packet directions or until light golden.

Step 4 :Divide the rice mixture and sausages among serving plates. Sprinkle with coriander. Serve with the yoghurt.

RECIPE NOTES

Allow for standing time.

SWAP ME: Currants add a touch of sweetness to this dish. If you can't find them, try sultanas or dried cranberries.

VEGAN GINGERBREAD

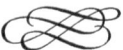

INGREDIENTS

- 2 tsp white chia seeds
- 1 1/2 cups plain flour, plus extra for dusting
- 1 tbsp ground ginger
- 1 tsp ground allspice
- 100g original Nuttelex spread
- 1/2 cup dark brown sugar
- 1 tbsp treacle
- EGG-FREE ROYAL ICING
- 1/2 cup pure icing sugar
- 1 tsp glucose syrup
- 1 tsp lemon juice

Step 1 :Place chia seeds and 1 1/2 tablespoons water in a small bowl. Stir to combine. Stand, stirring occasionally, for 20 minutes or until mixture has thickened.

Step 2 :Sift flour and spices into a large bowl. Add spread. Using your fingertips, rub spread into flour until mixture resembles fine crumbs. Add sugar, treacle and chia mixture. Stir until mixture just starts to 100 super food ideas DECEMBER 2018 What would Christmas be without gingerbread? Our version uses no egg or dairy, so whether you're making biscuits or a house, everyone can join in on the festivities GINGERBREAD come together. Turn out onto a lightly floured surface. Knead until smooth. Shape into 2 discs. Wrap each disc in plastic wrap. Refrigerate for 1 hour.

Step 3 :Preheat oven to 180C/160C fan-forced. Grease 2 large baking trays. Line with baking paper. Roll 1 dough disc out between 2 sheets of baking paper until 3mm thick. Using a 6.5cm gingerbread man and 6.5cm Christmas tree cookie cutter, cut shapes from dough, re-rolling and cutting trimmings (see note). Place 4cm apart, on prepared trays. Using a skewer, give the gingerbread men eyes and mouths.

Step 4 :Bake for 12 minutes or until edges start to brown. Stand on trays for 5 minutes. Transfer to a wire rack to cool. Repeat with remaining dough disc, using a 5cm gingerbread man and 5cm Christmas tree cookie cutter. Bake for 10 minutes or until edges start to brown.

Step 5 :Make Egg-free Royal Icing: Sift icing sugar into a bowl. Add 3/4 teaspoon water, glucose syrup and lemon juice. Stir until smooth. Spoon mixture into a piping bag fitted with a 2mm plain nozzle. Using the picture as a guide, decorate trees and men with icing. Stand overnight to set. Serve.

RECIPE NOTES

If the dough shapes are too soft to move once cut, place in the freezer for 10 minutes to firm.

VEGAN CARBONARA

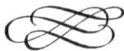

INGREDIENTS

- 1 tablespoon soy sauce
- 1 teaspoon smoked paprika
- 1/2 teaspoon garlic powder
- 1/2 teaspoon onion powder
- 1 tablespoon brown sugar
- 1/2 cup coconut flakes
- 300g silken tofu, chopped
- 1/4 cup nutritional yeast
- 1 tablespoon lemon juice
- 1/2 teaspoon sea salt
- 1/4 cup unsweetened almond milk
- 375g spaghetti (see note)
- 1 tablespoon extra virgin olive oil
- 1 brown onion, finely chopped
- 2 garlic cloves, crushed
- Roughly chopped fresh flat-leaf parsley leaves, to serve

METHOD

Step 1 :Preheat oven to 180C/160C fan-forced. Line a large baking tray with baking paper.

Step 2 :Combine soy sauce, paprika, garlic powder, onion powder and sugar in a bowl. Add coconut. Stir until well coated. Spoon onto prepared tray. Spread out to form a single layer. Bake, stirring halfway through, for 10 minutes or until coconut is golden. Set aside to cool (it will crisp on standing).

Step 3 :Meanwhile, place tofu, yeast, lemon juice, salt and almond milk in a food processor. Process until very smooth.

Step 4 :Cook pasta in a large saucepan of boiling water following packet directions. Drain, reserving 1/4 cup cooking liquid.

Step 5 :Heat oil in a large deep frying pan over medium-high heat. Add onion. Cook, stirring, for 5 minutes or until softened. Add crushed garlic. Cook for 30 seconds or until fragrant. Remove from heat. Add pasta, tofu mixture and reserved cooking liquid to pan. Toss until well combined. Add 3/4 of the coconut mixture. Gently toss to combine. Season with salt and pepper.

Step 6 :Divide pasta among serving bowls. Top with remaining coconut mixture. Sprinkle with parsley. Serve.

RECIPE NOTES

Many dried pasta varieties are egg-free, but always check the label on the pasta to ensure it is suitable for vegans.

VEGAN SCONES

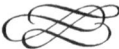

INGREDIENTS

- 2 x 400ml cans chilled coconut cream (see notes)
- 2 cups self-raising flour
- 1 tbsp caster sugar
- Pinch of salt
- 60g original Nuttelex spread
- 2 tsp icing sugar mixture
- 1/2 tsp vanilla bean paste
- Strawberry jam, to serve

METHOD

Step 1 :Preheat oven to 220C/200C fan-forced. Line a baking tray with baking paper.

Step 2 :Scoop the thick layer of coconut cream from each can of coconut cream and place in a bowl (about 1 cup). Cover with plastic wrap. Refrigerate. Sift flour, caster sugar and salt into a large bowl.

Add spread. Using fingertips, rub spread into flour mixture until mixture resembles fine breadcrumbs. Make a well in centre of mixture. Add ¾ cup remaining coconut cream liquid to well. Using a flat-bladed knife, stir until a sticky dough forms. Turn out onto a lightly floured surface. Knead gently until just smooth. Reserve 1 tablespoon remaining coconut cream liquid (see notes).

Step 3 :Using a lightly floured rolling pin, gently roll dough out until 2cm-thick. Using a 6cm round cutter, cut out rounds. Press leftover dough together. Repeat to make 12 rounds. Place, just touching, on prepared tray. Brush with reserved coconut cream liquid. Bake for 12 to 15 minutes or until golden and hollow when tapped on top.

Step 4 :Using a whisk, whisk reserved chilled coconut cream, icing sugar and vanilla until soft peaks form. Serve scones with jam and coconut cream mixture.

RECIPE NOTES

Refrigerate cans of coconut cream overnight (do not shake) before beginning recipe.

Store remaining coconut cream in an airtight container in the fridge for up to 2 days.

VEGAN GINGERBREAD DOUGHNUTS

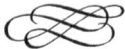

INGREDIENTS

- 310ml (1 1/4 cups) unsweetened almond milk
- 2 teaspoons apple cider vinegar
- 60g (1/3 cup) coconut sugar
- 100g vegan olive oil spread
- 2 1/2 tablespoons treacle
- 1 teaspoon vanilla extract
- 300g (2 cups) wholemeal spelt flour
- 3 teaspoons ground ginger
- 2 teaspoons ground cinnamon
- 1 teaspoon ground allspice
- 1 teaspoon baking powder
- 1/4 teaspoon bicarbonate of soda
- 120g pure icing sugar, sifted
- 3-4 teaspoons fresh lemon juice
- Freeze-dried strawberries, crushed, to decorate

METHOD

Step 1 :Preheat the oven to 180C/160C fan forced. Lightly spray 12 holes of a 7cm-diameter doughnut pan with oil. Combine almond milk and vinegar in a jug. Set aside for 5 minutes.

Step 2 :Use electric beaters to beat the coconut sugar, olive oil spread, treacle and vanilla in a large bowl for 2 minutes or until thick and creamy.

Step 3 :Sift the flour, ginger, cinnamon, allspice, baking powder and bicarb into a bowl. Fold the flour and milk mixtures, in alternating batches, into the coconut sugar mixture until just combined.

Step 4 :Divide the mixture among prepared doughnut holes. Bake for 15 minutes or until the doughnuts are golden and a skewer inserted into the doughnut comes out clean. Set aside for 2-3 minutes to cool slightly before turning onto a wire rack to cool completely.

Step 5 :Combine the icing sugar and enough lemon juice in a bowl until smooth, thick and a spreadable consistency. Spread over the top of the doughnuts. Sprinkle with freeze-dried strawberries before the icing sets.

RECIPE NOTES

Find freeze-dried strawberries in the health food aisle at the supermarket. Add to muffins or scatter over breakfast cereal or muesli.

VEGAN ZUCCHINI FRITTERS

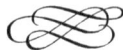

INGREDIENTS

- 4 (about 600g) medium zucchini
- 1 1/2 tablespoons flaxseed meal
- 2 teaspoons olive oil, plus extra, to shallow-fry
- 3 green shallots, thinly sliced
- 2 garlic cloves, finely chopped
- 55g (1/2 cup) finely grated vegan cheese
- 75g (1/2 cup) self-raising flour
- Pinch cayenne pepper
- Cherry tomatoes, halved, to serve
- Fresh mint leaves, to serve
- Thinly sliced red onion, to serve
- Olive oil, to drizzle

METHOD

Step 1 :Coarsely grate the zucchini. Transfer to a colander. Season and toss to combine. Set aside for 5 minutes. Take handfuls of zucchini and squeeze out as much liquid as possible. Transfer to a large mixing bowl.

Step 2 :Place the flaxseed and 80ml (1/3 cup) water in a small bowl. Stir to combine. Set aside.

Step 3 :Heat the oil in a non-stick frying pan over high heat. Add the shallot and garlic and cook, stirring often, for 2 minutes or until soft. Add to the zucchini, along with the flaxseed mixture and the cheese. Sift over the flour and add the cayenne. Mix until well combined.

Step 4 :Pour enough oil in a non-stick frying pan to come 3mm up the side and place over medium heat. Drop 1/4 cups of mixture into the oil and spread out to approximately 8cm rounds. Cook, turning halfway, for 3 minutes or until golden and cooked through. Transfer to a plate lined with paper towel. Repeat with remaining mixture to make 8 fritters. Season and serve with the tomato, mint, onion drizzled with olive oil.

VEGAN PESTO GNOCCHI

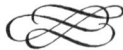

INGREDIENTS

- 2 corncobs
- 80ml (1/3 cup) extra virgin olive oil
- 1 leek, trimmed, thinly sliced
- 3 garlic cloves, finely chopped
- 320g pkt Mix-a-Mato Tomatoes, larger ones halved
- 2 zucchini, sliced
- Pinch of dried chilli flakes (optional)
- 500g packet vegan potato gnocchi
- 200g packet vegan basil pesto
- Fresh basil leaves, to serve

METHOD

Step 1 :Heat a chargrill pan on high heat. Lightly brush the corn with some of the oil. Grill the corn, turning often, for 10 minutes or until charred. Set aside for 3 minutes to cool slightly. Use a sharp knife to cut down the length of the cob close to the core to remove the kernels.

Step 2 :Meanwhile, heat 1 tablespoon remaining oil in a large non-stick frying pan over high heat. Add the leek and garlic. Cook, stirring often, for 2 minutes or until the leek has softened slightly. Add the remaining oil, tomato, zucchini and chilli, if using. Reduce heat to medium and cook, stirring occasionally, for 10 minutes or until the tomato has collapsed. Season well.

Step 3 :While the sauce is simmering, cook the gnocchi in a large saucepan of boiling water following packet directions (see tip). Drain and return gnocchi to the pan.

Step 4 :Add the tomato mixture and pesto to the gnocchi. Gently toss to combine then serve topped with fresh basil.

RECIPE NOTES

Keep the water for the gnocchi at a light boil, if you can. A gentler cooking process will only add an extra 30 seconds or so and is less likely to break up the gnocchi.

VEGAN MUSHROOM BOURGUIGNON

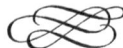

INGREDIENTS

- 10g dried porcini mushrooms
- 160ml (2/3 cup) Massel vegetable liquid stock, warmed
- 80ml (1/3 cup) extra virgin olive oil
- 300g cap mushrooms, thickly sliced
- 300g button mushrooms, thickly sliced
- 200g (about 8-10) French shallots, peeled, halved
- 2 carrots, peeled, thickly sliced
- 2 garlic cloves, crushed
- 1 tbsp tomato paste
- 2 tsp plain flour
- 80ml (1/3 cup) red wine
- 2 fresh thyme sprigs, leaves finely chopped
- 1kg brushed potatoes, peeled, cut into 3-4cm pieces
- Continental parsley sprigs, to serve

METHOD

Step 1 :Place the porcini mushrooms in a heatproof bowl then pour over the stock. Set aside to soak until required.

Step 2 :Heat 2 teaspoons of the oil in a large, deep frying pan over high heat. Add one-third of the cap and button mushrooms and cook, stirring occasionally, for 2-3 minutes or until the mushrooms start to soften. Transfer to a bowl. Repeat with the remaining mushrooms, in 2 more batches, adding 2 more teaspoons of oil to each batch.

Step 3 :Add 1 tablespoon of the remaining oil to the pan and reduce heat to medium. Add the shallot and carrot. Cook, stirring often, for 5 minutes or until starts to soften. Add the garlic and cook, stirring, for 30 seconds or until aromatic. Add the tomato paste and stir to coat. Add the flour and cook, stirring, for 2 minutes. Add the wine, thyme, porcini and soaking liquid. Stir to combine. Reduce heat to low. Cover and simmer, stirring occasionally, for 10-15 minutes or until the vegetables are soft.

Step 4 :Meanwhile, cook the potato in a large saucepan of boiling water for 10 minutes or until tender. Drain and mash. For super smooth mash, push through a sieve. Season and stir in remaining 1 1/2 tablespoons of oil.

Step 5 :Return the mushrooms and their juices to the frying pan and cook, covered, for 5 minutes or until the mushrooms are soft. Season. Serve the mushroom bourguignon with the mash, sprinkled with parsley.

VEGAN BUFFALO WINGS

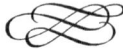

INGREDIENTS

- 1 cup self-raising flour
- 1/4 cup cornflour
- 2 tsp garlic powder
- 1 1/2 tsp sweet paprika
- 1 tsp sea salt
- 1 1/4 cups chilled soda water
- Vegetable oil, for deep-frying
- 1.4kg cauliflower, trimmed, cut into small florets
- 3/4 cup maple syrup
- 2 tbsp Sriracha chilli sauce
- EGG-FREE AIOLI
- 125g can chickpeas
- 1/2 tsp garlic powder
- 1 tsp Dijon mustard
- 2 tsp white wine vinegar
- 1/2 cup vegetable oil
- 1 tbsp finely chopped fresh chives
- Select all ingredients

METHOD

Step 1 :Make Egg-free Aioli: Drain chickpeas, reserving liquid. Place garlic powder, mustard, vinegar, 8 chickpeas and reserved chickpea liquid in a small food processor (see note). Process until smooth. With motor operating, gradually add oil in a slow, steady stream until light and creamy. Transfer to a small serving bowl. Stir in chives and season with salt and pepper.

Step 2 :Place flour, cornflour, garlic powder, paprika and salt in a large bowl. Whisk to combine. Make a well in centre. Slowly pour in soda water, whisking to form a smooth batter.

Step 3 :Pour enough oil in a large saucepan until 1/3 full. Heat over medium-high heat until hot. Working in batches, dip cauliflower in batter, allowing excess to drain off. Add to oil. Cook cauliflower for 3 minutes or until golden. Using a slotted spoon, transfer cauliflower to a large wire rack set over a large baking tray to drain. Repeat with remaining cauliflower and batter.

Step 4 :Combine maple syrup and chilli sauce in a small saucepan over medium heat. Cook, stirring occasionally, for 3 minutes or until simmering. Simmer for 30 seconds. Remove from heat.

Step 5 :Working quickly, place cauliflower in a large heatproof bowl. Pour over sauce mixture. Toss to coat. Transfer to a serving dish. Serve immediately with aioli.

RECIPE NOTES

Store remaining chickpeas in an airtight container in the fridge for up to 3 days.

VEGAN INDIAN CURRY

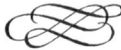

INGREDIENTS

- 1 tbs vegetable oil
- 200g tempeh, cut into 2cm pieces
- 1 brown onion, finely chopped
- 2 celery sticks, finely chopped
- 2 carrots, peeled, finely chopped
- 2 garlic cloves, crushed
- 120g (1/2 cup) yellow curry paste (see tip)
- 2 x 420g cans chickpeas, rinsed, drained
- 500ml (2 cups) So Good Cashew Unsweetened milk
- 400ml can coconut cream
- 6 silverbeet leaves, stalk trimmed, leaves shredded
- Steamed brown rice, to serve
- 1 long fresh red chilli, chopped
- 80g (1/2 cup) roasted cashews, chopped
- 1 tbs nigella seeds (optional)
- Fresh basil leaves, to serve
- Pappadums, to serve

METHOD

Step 1 :Heat oil in a large saucepan over mediumhigh heat. Cook tempeh, turning occasionally, for 3 minutes or until browned. Transfer to a plate lined with paper towel to drain.

Step 2 :Add onion, celery, carrot and garlic. Stir often for 3 minutes or until softened slightly. Stir in paste until aromatic then chickpeas.

Step 3 :Pour milk and coconut cream into pan. Bring to the boil. Reduce heat to medium. Simmer for 3 minutes or until sauce thickens slightly. Stir in silverbeet. Cook for 2 minutes or until just wilted. Remove from heat and season.

Step 4 :Divide rice and curry among serving plates. Top with tempeh, chilli, cashew, nigella seeds, if using, and basil. Serve with pappadums

VEGAN SPINACH AND FETTA PIE

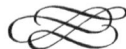

INGREDIENTS

- 4 bunches English spinach, stems trimmed, leaves chopped
- 1 tbs olive oil
- 3 spring onions, thinly sliced
- 2 garlic cloves, crushed
- 2 tbs pine nuts, toasted
- 120g vegan fetta, crumbled
- 200g Chris' Plant Based Spring Onion dip
- 2 tbs chopped dill
- 2 tsp finely grated lemon rind
- 16 sheets filo pastry
- 1 tbs sesame seeds
- Garden salad, to serve

- 20cm x 30cm (base measurement) slice pan

METHOD

Step 1 :Preheat oven to 200°C. Spray a 20cm x 30cm (base measurement) slice pan with olive oil spray. Rinse spinach in cold water. Place, with water clinging, in a saucepan over medium-high heat. Cook, stirring, for 2-3 mins or until spinach wilts. Transfer to a colander. Cool slightly. Squeeze out excess liquid. Set aside to cool.

Step 2 :Heat oil in a frying pan over medium heat. Add spring onion and garlic. Cook, stirring, for 2 mins or until spring onion softens. Transfer to a bowl. Stir in spinach, pine nuts, fetta, dip, dill and lemon rind. Season with pepper.

Step 3 :Place pastry sheets on a clean work surface and cover with a damp tea towel. Spray 1 sheet with olive oil spray. Top with another sheet. Spray with olive oil spray. Repeat with 6 more pastry sheets to make a stack. Repeat with olive oil spray and remaining pastry sheets to make another stack. Place 1 pastry stack in the prepared pan, trimming to fit. Spread spinach filling over the pastry in pan. Top with remaining pastry stack. Fold in excess pastry. Score the top with a small sharp knife. Spray with olive oil spray. Sprinkle with sesame seeds.

Step 4 :Bake for 25-30 mins or until golden. Cool for 5 mins. Cut into slices. Serve with salad.

TARTE TATIN TOMATO VEGAN

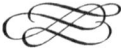

INGREDIENTS

- 145g (1 cup) raw cashews
- 800g tomato medley mix
- 3/4 cup fresh basil leaves, plus extra, to serve
- 1 tablespoon fresh lemon juice
- 1-2 teaspoon nutritional yeast, to taste
- 1 tablespoon balsamic vinegar
- 1 tablespoon pure maple syrup
- 8 small fresh thyme sprigs
- 1 sheet frozen reduced-fat vegan puff pastry, just thawed
- Baby rocket, to serve (optional)

METHOD

Step 1 : Place cashews in bowl. Cover with water. Leave overnight to soak.

Step 2 : Preheat oven to 150°C/130°C fan forced. Line a large baking

VEGAN RECIPES

tray with baking paper. Place tomatoes on tray. Spray with oil. Bake for 1 1/2 hours or until softened. Press lightly to remove excess juice.

Step 3 :Meanwhile, drain cashews. Place basil in blender. Process until finely chopped. Add cashews, lemon juice and 80ml (1/3 cup) water. Blend, occasionally scraping down side of jug, for 2-3 minutes or until thick and smooth. Add nutritional yeast. Season. Blend until combined.

Step 4 :Increase oven to 210°C/190°C fan forced. Lightly spray a 22cm (base measurement) ovenproof frying pan with oil. Add vinegar and maple syrup. Simmer over a high heat for 1-2 minutes or until the mixture thickens and coats base of the pan. Remove from heat.

Step 5 :Sprinkle thyme over syrup mixture. Carefully arrange tomatoes snugly over the top, leaving any juices on the tray. Place the pastry over top, tucking in edges as needed. Bake for 20-25 minutes or until pastry is golden. Set aside for 2-3 minutes to cool slightly.

Step 6 :Place a plate on top of pastry. Carefully invert. Sprinkle with extra basil. Drizzle over half the pesto cream. Serve with rocket,

VEGAN CUPCAKES WITH CARAMEL POPCORN

INGREDIENTS

- 1 1/3 cups (200g) plain flour
- 1 1/2 tsp baking powder
- 1/2 tsp bicarbonate of soda
- 190g caster sugar
- 2/3 cup (160ml) almond milk
- 300g Flora Plant Original
- 3 tsp vanilla extract
- 1 1/4 cups (200g) icing sugar mixture
- 2 tbs golden syrup
- 3 cups popped popcorn
- 4 tbs sprinkles
- 1/3-cup (80ml) muffin pan
- Paper cases

METHOD

Step 1 :Preheat oven to 180°C. Line 8 holes of a 1/3-cup (80ml) muffin pan with paper cases. Sift the flour, baking powder and bicarbonate of soda into a medium bowl. Stir in 1/2 cup (110g) caster sugar. Add the milk, 100g of the Flora Plant Original and 2 tsp vanilla. Whisk until smooth. Spoon evenly among the paper cases. Bake for 20-25 mins or until a skewer inserted in the centres comes out clean. Transfer to a wire rack to cool completely.

Step 2 :Use an electric mixer to beat the icing sugar, 125g of the remaining Flora Plant Original and the remaining vanilla in a bowl until pale and smooth. Transfer to a piping bag fitted with a 1cm fluted nozzle.

Step 3 :Line a baking tray with baking paper. Place golden syrup, remaining caster sugar and remaining Flora Plant Original in a saucepan over medium heat. Bring to the boil. Reduce heat to low. Cook for 5 mins or until mixture thickens. Remove from heat. Stir in popcorn and 2 tbs sprinkles. Cool slightly. Divide the mixture into 8 portions. Shape into balls. Place on lined tray to set.

Step 4 :Pipe icing onto the cupcakes. Top with caramel popcorn and remaining sprinkles.

LEMON AND BLUEBERRY VEGAN TART

INGREDIENTS

- 1 1/1 cup (160g) whole almonds
- 2 cups (225g) cashews
- 1/4 cup (35g) pistachios
- 1/2 cup (40g) shredded coconut
- Pinch of salt
- 12 fresh dates, pitted, chopped
- 270ml can coconut cream
- 1 lemon, rind finely grated, juiced
- 1/3 cup (80ml) maple syrup
- Pinch of ground turmeric
- Blueberries, to decorate
- Thyme sprigs, to decorate
- CANDIED LEMON
- 2 lemons, thinly sliced
- 1/2 cup (110g) caster sugar

METHOD

Step 1 :Place the cashews in a large bowl. Pour over enough boiling water to cover. Set aside for 4 hours to soak.

Step 2 :Lightly grease a 24cm (base measurement) fluted tart tin with removable base. Line the base with baking paper. Place on a baking tray.

Step 3 :Place almonds, pistachios, shredded coconut and salt in a food processor. Process until finely chopped. Add dates and process until very finely chopped and mixture holds together when pinched. Spoon into prepared tin. Use the back of a metal spoon to push the mixture evenly over base and side of the tin. Place in the freezer to set.

Step 4 :Drain the cashews and place in a blender. Add coconut cream, lemon rind, lemon juice and maple syrup. Blend until very smooth and creamy. Add turmeric and blend until smooth. Pour into the tart case in tin. Gently tap on the bench to smooth the surface. Place in freezer for 2 hours or until firm.

Step 5 :Meanwhile, to make the candied lemon, line a baking tray with baking paper. Place lemon, sugar and 1 1/2 cups (375ml) water in a frying pan. Bring to a simmer over medium heat. Cook, turning lemon occasionally, for 20 mins or until rind is translucent. Transfer the lemon to the lined tray. Increase heat to medium-high. Bring syrup in the pan to the boil. Cook for 3-5 mins or until syrup thickens. Set aside to cool completely.

Step 6 :Transfer tart to a serving plate. Top with candied lemon, blueberries and thyme. Drizzle with the lemon syrup.

VEGAN SPINACH FILO SCROLL

INGREDIENTS

- 1 1/2 tbs olive oil
- 5 spring onions, thinly sliced
- 2 garlic cloves, crushed
- 2 x 280g pkts Coles Australian Baby Spinach
- 300g Coles Nature's Kitchen Silken Tofu, drained, crumbled
- 1/3 cup (25g) panko breadcrumbs
- 1 1/2 tbs nutritional yeast seasoning
- 10g chopped dill
- 1 tbs finely grated lemon rind
- 15 sheets filo pastry
- 2 tsp sesame seeds
- 250g vine-ripened cherry tomatoes
- 2 large baking trays with baking paper

METHOD

Step 1 :Preheat oven to 200°C. Line 2 large baking trays with baking paper. Heat 2 tsp of oil in a large, deep frying pan over medium heat. Cook spring onion and garlic, stirring, for 2-3 mins or until spring onion softens. Transfer to a plate.

Step 2 :Heat 1 tsp of the remaining oil in the pan and add one-quarter of the spinach. Cook, tossing, for 2 mins or until spinach wilts. Transfer to a large bowl. Repeat, in 3 more batches, with remaining oil and spinach. Set aside to cool slightly. Use your hands to squeeze as much liquid from the spinach as possible. Discard the liquid.

Step 3 :Combine the spinach, spring onion mixture, tofu, breadcrumbs, nutritional yeast seasoning, dill and lemon rind in a large bowl. Season.

Step 4 :Place the pastry sheets on a clean work surface. Cover with a damp tea towel. Spray 1 sheet with olive oil spray. Top with another sheet and spray with olive oil spray. Top with 1 more sheet and spray with oil. Spoon one-fifth of the spinach mixture along 1 long edge of the stack, leaving a 3cm gap at each end. Roll up to enclose the filling. Arrange, seam-side down, in a coil in the centre of 1 of the lined trays. Repeat with the remaining pastry sheets and spinach mixture to make 4 more rolls. Arrange rolls, seam-side down, on tray to form a coil. Spray with olive oil spray and sprinkle with sesame seeds.

Step 5 :Place the tomatoes on the remaining lined tray. Spray with olive oil spray. Bake the pastry and tomatoes for 20 mins or until the tomatoes begin to collapse. Transfer the tomatoes to a plate. Cook the pastry for a further 15 mins or until golden brown. Set aside for 10 mins to cool slightly. Cut into wedges and serve with the tomatoes.

RECIPE NOTES

Allow for cooling time.

VEGAN CHOCOLATE LAVA CAKES

INGREDIENTS

- 80g (1/2 cup) wholemeal spelt flour
- 2 1/2 tablespoons cocoa powder
- 1 teaspoon baking powder
- 1/4 teaspoon bicarbonate of soda
- 30g (1/4 cup) almond meal
- 150g cooked sweet potato, mashed, cooled
- 60g (1/3 cup) coconut sugar
- 2 tablespoons macadamia oil
- 2 teaspoons vanilla extract
- 125ml (1/2 cup) unsweetened almond milk
- 75g vegan dark chocolate, cut into 12 pieces
- Vegan vanilla ice-cream or coconut yoghurt, to serve (optional)

METHOD

Step 1 :Preheat the oven to 190C/170C fan forced. Lightly grease six 125ml (1/2 cup) ramekins with oil spray. Line the bases with baking paper.

Step 2 :Sift the flour, cocoa, baking powder and bicarb into a bowl. Add the almond meal and stir to combine.

Step 3 :Use electric beaters to beat the sweet potato, sugar, oil and vanilla in a large bowl until thick and smooth. Add the flour mixture and milk, in alternating batches, beginning and ending with the flour mixture, until just combined.

Step 4 :Divide the mixture among the prepared ramekins. Place 2 pieces of chocolate into the centre of each. Push chocolate one-third of the way into the mixture. Bake for 10 minutes or until cakes are just firm to the touch (do not overcook). Set aside for 1-2 minutes to cool slightly.

Step 5 :Gently turn the cakes onto serving plates. Serve topped with coconut yoghurt or vegan ice-cream, if using.

VEGAN MANGO JELLY SLICE

INGREDIENTS

- 4 Weet-Bix
- 80g (1/2 cup) wholemeal spelt flour
- 65g (3/4 cup) desiccated coconut
- 50g (1/4 cup) coconut sugar
- 1 1/2 tsp ground cinnamon
- 1 tsp baking powder
- 90g Nuttelex Olive spread, melted
- Fresh passionfruit pulp, to serve (optional)
- CUSTARD
- 35g (1/4 cup) cornflour
- 250ml (1 cup) canned coconut milk
- 250ml (1 cup) unsweetened almond and coconut milk
- 2 tbsp pure maple syrup
- 3 tsp vanilla bean paste
- MANGO JELLY
- 185ml (3/4 cup) cold water
- 400g frozen mango, thawed
- 2 tbsp pure maple syrup

- 1 1/2 tbsp fresh lime juice
- 1 Jel-It-In Vegetarian gelling powder

METHOD

Step 1 :Preheat oven to 180°C/160°C fan forced. Grease and line base and sides of a 16 x 26cm slice pan with baking paper, allowing the paper to slightly overhang the long sides.

Step 2 :Place the Weet-Bix, flour, coconut, sugar, cinnamon and baking powder in a food processor. Process until resembles fine crumbs. Add the Nuttelex. Process until well combined. Press the mixture firmly over the base of prepared pan. Bake for 12 minutes or until light golden. Set aside to cool.

Step 3 :Meanwhile, to make the custard, combine cornflour and 80ml (1/3 cup) coconut milk in a saucepan until smooth. Stir in almond and coconut milk, maple syrup, vanilla and remaining coconut milk until combined. Stir over medium heat for 5 minutes or until thickens and coats back of a spoon. Quickly spread evenly over base. Cover surface of custard with plastic wrap. Set aside to cool to room temperature. Place in fridge to set.

Step 4 :To make mango jelly, combine Jel-It-In and cold water in a small bowl until dissolves. Process mango, maple syrup, lime juice and gelatine mixture in food processor until smooth. Transfer to a saucepan over medium heat. Stir constantly for 3-4 minutes or until comes to the boil. Simmer for 1-2 minutes or until thickens. Working quickly, evenly pour jelly over top of the custard. Set aside to cool slightly. Cover and place in the fridge until set.

Step 5 :Top the slice with passionfruit, if using. Cut into pieces to serve.

VEGAN CHOC MOUSSE EGGS

INGREDIENTS

- 250g fresh medjool dates, pitted
- 65g (3/4 cup) desiccated coconut
- 125g (1/2 cup) walnuts
- 2 tbsp dark cocoa powder, plus 30g (1/4 cup), extra
- 2 ripe avocados
- 60ml (1/4 cup) pure maple syrup
- 2 tsp vanilla extract
- Pistachio kernels, finely chopped, to decorate
- Freeze-dried strawberries, finely chopped, to decorate

METHOD

Step 1 : Place date, coconut, walnuts and cocoa in a food processor and process until the mixture is finely chopped and comes together. Divide into 24 portions and roll into egg-shaped balls. Place in the fridge for 1 hour to chill.

Step 2 :Meanwhile, clean the food processor bowl then place the avocado, maple syrup, vanilla, extra cocoa and a generous pinch of salt. Process until smooth. Transfer to a bowl and place in the fridge for 1 hour to chill.

Step 3 :Use your thumb to make a deep indentation in each egg. Spoon the mousse into a piping bag fitted with a 1cm fluted nozzle. Pipe the mousse into the indents. Sprinkle with pistachio or strawberry.

VEGAN LEMON TARTS

INGREDIENTS

- 270ml can coconut cream
- 80ml (1/3 cup) lemon juice
- 2 teaspoons finely grated lemon rind
- 1 1/2 tablespoons cornflour
- 2 tablespoons icing sugar
- Pinch ground turmeric
- Finely chopped pistachios, to serve
- Finely chopped lemon, to serve (optional)
- Finely chopped lime, to serve (optional)
- PASTRY
- 225g (1 1/2 cups) plain flour
- 1 tablespoon icing sugar mixture
- Pinch salt
- 45g (1/2 cup) desiccated coconut
- 170g (3/4 cup) solidified coconut oil, chilled
- 1 teaspoon vanilla essence
- 1 1/2 tablespoons iced water

METHOD

Step 1 :To make the pastry, sift the flour, icing sugar and salt into a medium bowl. Stir in the coconut. Use a teaspoon to scoop the coconut oil into small pieces and add to the bowl. Use your fingertips to rub the coconut oil into the flour until the mixture resembles coarse breadcrumbs. Add the vanilla and water, and use a knife to mix until a dough forms, adding another 2 teaspoons of iced water if necessary.

Step 2 :Gently knead the dough and divide into 6 equal portions. Roll out a portion between 2 sheets of baking paper large enough to fit an 8.5cm (base measurement) loose-based tart tin. Transfer pastry to the tin and gently press in. Trim overhanging pastry. Use your thumb to gently press the pastry around the side so it reaches about 3mm above the edge of the tin. Repeat with remaining pastry to line 5 more tins. Place in the fridge for 30 minutes to chill.

Step 3 :Preheat oven to 180C/160C fan forced. Place tins on a baking tray and bake for 20 minutes or until light golden. Set aside to cool completely.

Step 4 :Meanwhile, combine the coconut cream, lemon juice and rind in a small saucepan. Place the cornflour in a small bowl. Add about 2 tablespoons of the coconut cream mixture to the bowl and stir until smooth. Add to the saucepan along with the icing sugar and stir to combine. Add the turmeric. Use a balloon whisk to gently whisk over low heat for 3 minutes or until the mixture boils and thickens, making sure it doesn't stick to the bottom of the pan. Transfer mixture to a heatproof bowl and set aside, stirring often, for about 20 minutes, to cool. Cover the surface with plastic wrap and place in the fridge for 30 minutes or until chilled.

Step 5 :the filling and divide among the cooked tart shells. Smooth the surface. Top with pistachios and chopped lemon and lime, if using.

. . .

RECIPE NOTES

When making the pastry, try to keep everything quite cool, so the pastry stays firm. If it seems to be too soft when rolling out, place in fridge briefly.

The turmeric is simply to add colour to the filling. To get a "pinch", use the tip of a small pointed knife to lift a tiny bit from the jar. The colour will become stronger as it cools.

VEGAN QUINOA PILAF

INGREDIENTS

- 1 tablespoon extra virgin olive oil
- 1 brown onion, finely chopped
- 2 garlic cloves, crushed
- 200g (1 cup) quinoa, rinsed, drained
- 500ml (2 cups) Massel Salt Reduced Vegetable Stock Cubes
- 1 bunch broccolini, cut into 3cm pieces, stalks halved if large
- 1 large corncob, kernels removed
- 1 bunch asparagus, trimmed, sliced lengthways
- 150g sugar snap peas, halved lengthways
- 100g baby spinach
- 2 tablespoob chopped unsalted pistachio kernels
- 2 tablespoon pomegranate arils
- Fresh lime wedges, to serve

METHOD

Step 1 :Heat the oil in a large saucepan over high heat. Cook onion, stirring occasionally, for 5 minutes or until softened. Add garlic and cook, stirring, for 1 minute or until aromatic.

Step 2 :Add quinoa and stock. Bring to boil. Reduce heat to low. Cover and simmer for 12 minutes or until almost all stock is absorbed. Add the broccolini, corn, asparagus and peas. Stir to combine. Cover and cook for 2 minutes or until all stock is absorbed. Remove from heat. Set aside, covered, for 3-4 minutes to steam.

Step 3 :Stir through the spinach and season. Sprinkle the pilaf with the pistachios and pomegranate arils. Serve with lime wedges.

VEGAN OREO CUPCAKES

INGREDIENTS

- 4 x 23g packets mini Oreo cookies
- 1 1/3 cups self-raising flour
- 1/3 cup Dutch-processed cocoa powder
- 1/2 cup brown sugar
- 2 x 120g tubs apple puree
- 1/3 cup vegetable oil
- 1 teaspoon vanilla extract
- 1/3 cup soy milk
- 1 teaspoon bicarbonate of soda
- 1 tablespoon apple cider vinegar
- CHOCOLATE FROSTING
- 250g Nuttelex original dairy-free spread
- 1 teaspoon vanilla extract
- 2 2/3 cups icing sugar mixture
- 1/3 cup Dutch-processed cocoa powder, sifted

METHOD

Step 1 :Preheat oven to 180C/160C fan-forced. Line a 12-hole (1/3-cup-capacity) muffin pan with paper cases.

Step 2 :Reserve 14 Oreo cookies. Roughly chop remaining cookies. Sift flour and cocoa into a large bowl. Add sugar and chopped cookies. Stir until well combined. Make a well. Add apple puree, oil and vanilla to well, without stirring. Place milk in a jug. Add bicarbonate of soda, then vinegar. Lightly whisk with a fork until frothy. Add to well. Stir until mixture is just combined.

Step 3 :Divide mixture evenly among prepared pan holes. Bake for 15 to 17 minutes or until cakes spring back when lightly touched. Stand in pan for 5 minutes. Transfer to a wire rack to cool completely.

Step 4 :Make Chocolate Frosting. Using an electric mixer, beat Nuttelex, vanilla, icing sugar mixture and cocoa until light and fluffy. Spoon chocolate frosting into a piping bag fitted with a 1.5cm fluted nozzle.

Step 5 :Remove and discard icing from 2 of reserved cookies. Finely chop to coarse crumbs. Pipe frosting onto cupcakes. Top with remaining reserved cookies. Sprinkle with cookie crumbs. Serve.

VEGAN BURGER IN A LETTUCE BUN

INGREDIENTS

- 4 Herb & Sons Beef Burgers
- 250g cooked baby beetroot†, drained, chopped
- 2 tsp tahini
- 1 tsp ground cumin
- 2 small iceberg lettuces
- 2 tbs vegan mayonnaise
- 1 Lebanese cucumber, peeled into ribbons
- 2 radishes, thinly sliced
- Mint leaves, to serve

METHOD

Step 1 :Heat a chargrill on medium-high. Lightly spray burger patties with olive oil spray. Cook for 4-5 mins each side or until charred and heated through.

Step 2 :Meanwhile, place the beetroot, tahini and cumin in a food processor and process until smooth. Season.

Step 3 :Use a large serrated knife to cut 4cm-thick cheeks off each lettuce to make 8 buns.

Step 4 :Divide half the lettuce among serving plates. Top with the burger patties, mayonnaise, beetroot mixture, cucumber and radish. Sprinkle with mint leaves and top with the remaining lettuce. Serve immediately.

VEGAN ROASTED CAULIFLOWER SALAD

INGREDIENTS

- 1.2kg cauliflower, cut into small florets
- 185ml (3/4 cup) vegan buffalo wing sauce
- 150g mixed salad leaves
- 2 Lebanese cucumbers, thinly sliced
- 1 Delcado Hass avocado, cut into wedges
- 95g (1 cup) bought lightly salted roast chickpeas, coarsely chopped
- RANCH DRESSING
- 125ml (1/2 cup) vegan aïoli
- 1 teaspoon chopped fresh dill, plus extra, to serve

METHOD

Step 1:ROAST THE CAULIFLOWER Preheat oven to 220C/200C fan forced. Place the cauliflower and half the buffalo sauce on a large baking tray and toss to coat. Roast, turning once, for 20-25 minutes or until tender.

Step 2 :MAKE THE DRESSING To make ranch dressing, place aïoli, dill and 1 tbs water in a bowl and whisk until smooth.

Step 3 :TIME TO SERVE Pour the remaining buffalo sauce over the roasted cauliflower and toss to coat. Arrange the buffalo cauliflower, salad leaves and cucumber on a large serving dish. Drizzle over half the dressing. Top with avocado, chickpeas, extra dill and serve with remaining ranch dressing.

RECIPE NOTES

Time saver! Use frozen cauliflower florets to save on prep time. Roast straight from frozen. It's also an easy no-waste option, as you can weigh out the exact amount you need.

VEGAN CHOC-CHIP COOKIES

INGREDIENTS

- 110g Nuttelex vegan olive oil spread
- 150g (3/4 cup) coconut sugar
- 1 teaspoon pure vanilla extract
- 235g (1 1/2 cups) wholemeal spelt flour
- 1 teaspoon ground cinnamon
- 60ml (1/4 cup) unsweetened almond milk
- 80g vegan milk chocolate, chopped

METHOD

Step 1 :Preheat oven 180C/160C fan forced. Line a large baking tray with baking paper. Use electric beaters to beat the spread, sugar and vanilla in a bowl until pale and creamy.

Step 2 :Sift the flour and cinnamon into the spread mixture. Add the milk and chocolate. Stir until well combined and a soft sticky dough forms.

Step 3 :Use slightly wetted hands to roll tablespoonfuls of the mixture into balls. Place on the prepared tray, about 5cm apart. Flatten well with a fork. Bake for 12 minutes or until golden. Transfer to a wire rack to cool completely.

RECIPE NOTES

These cookies will keep for up to 3 days in an airtight container, but will soften slightly. They also freeze beautifully wrapped in plastic wrap.

ULTIMATE VEGAN BREAKFAST WRAP

INGREDIENTS

- 125g can black beans, rinsed, drained
- Pinch of dried chilli flakes
- 2 tsp fresh lemon juice
- 40g wholegrain wrap
- 20g baby spinach
- 1 roma tomato, sliced
- 1/4 avocado, sliced
- 2 tbsp fresh basil leaves
- Lemon wedge, to serve

METHOD

Step 1 :Coarsely mash the beans in a bowl. Stir in chilli and juice. Season.

Step 2 :Spread bean mixture over wrap. Top with the spinach, tomato, avocado and basil. Serve with lemon wedge, if using.

. . .

RECIPE NOTES

If you prefer your wrap toasted, fold over wrap to enclose and toast in a sandwich press until golden and crisp.

EASY VEGAN BOLOGNAISE

INGREDIENTS

- 375g Cucina Matese Fusilli
- 200g Coles Sliced Cup Mushrooms
- 400g can Coles Lentils, rinsed, drained,
- 425g Coles Nature's Kitchen Veggie Pasta Sauce
- 2 tbs finely chopped basil leaves
- Basil leaves, extra, to serve

METHOD

Step 1 :Cook the pasta in a saucepan of boiling water following packet directions or until al dente. Drain. Return to the pan.

Step 2 :Meanwhile, heat a large non-stick frying pan over high heat. Add the mushroom and cook, stirring, for 5 mins or until the mushroom softens. Add the lentils and pasta sauce and cook, stirring, for 5 mins or until the mixture thickens slightly. Add the chopped basil and stir to combine.

Step 3 :Add half the mushroom mixture to the pasta in the saucepan. Stir until combined. Divide the pasta mixture among serving bowls. Top with the remaining mushroom mixture and sprinkle with basil leaves to serve.

LIME AND RASPBERRY VEGAN CHEESECAKE

INGREDIENTS

- 700g cashews
- 1/2 cup (80g) almond kernels
- 1/2 cup (40g) shredded coconut
- 8 fresh dates, pitted, chopped
- 1 tbs coconut oil, melted
- Pinch of salt
- 2 limes, rind finely grated, juiced
- 2 x 270ml cans coconut cream
- 1/2 cup (125ml) maple syrup
- 250g fresh or frozen raspberries

METHOD

Step 1 :Divide the cashews evenly among 2 heatproof bowls. Pour over enough boiling water to cover. Set aside for 4 hours to soak.

Step 2 :Grease a 20cm (base measurement) springform pan and line the base and side with baking paper.

Step 3 :Place the almonds and coconut in a food processor. Process until finely chopped. Add the date, coconut oil and salt. Process until mixture holds together when pinched. Spoon the almond mixture over base of prepared pan and use the back of the spoon to spread and press evenly over the base. Place in the freezer for 30 mins to set.

Step 4 :Meanwhile, drain 1 bowl of cashews and place in a blender. Add the lime rind, lime juice, half the coconut cream and half the maple syrup. Blend until very smooth and creamy. Pour over the almond mixture in the pan and smooth the surface. Place in the freezer for 30 mins or until firm.

Step 5 :Drain remaining bowl of cashews. Place in a clean blender with the raspberries, remaining coconut cream and remaining maple syrup. Blend until very smooth and creamy. Pour over lime layer in pan. Smooth the surface. Place in freezer for 4 hours or until firm. Store in freezer until ready to eat.

Step 6 :Before serving, remove cheesecake from freezer. Set aside for 30 mins to soften slightly. Transfer to a serving platter. Cut into wedges to serve.

RECIPE NOTES

Allow for 4 hours soaking, 5 hours freezing and 30 mins standing time.

*Always check the label to make sure you're using vegan ingredients.

SERVE WITH raspberries, mint leaves and lime zest.

FREEZE ME: Store any leftover cheesecake in an airtight container in the freezer for up to 3 months.

VEGAN PASTA NOURISH BOWL

INGREDIENTS

- 125g wholemeal spiral pasta (see notes)
- 150g sugar snap peas
- 150g snow peas, trimmed
- 1 tablespoon apple cider vinegar
- 1 teaspoon maple syrup
- 1/4 small red cabbage, finely shredded
- 1 tablespoon tahini
- 1 tablespoon fresh lemon juice
- 2 teaspoons extra virgin olive oil
- 1 large carrot, peeled, shredded
- 200g Japanese marinated tofu, sliced

METHOD

Step 1 :Cook pasta in a large saucepan of boiling water following packet instructions, adding the sugar snaps and snow peas in the last minute of cooking. Drain and refresh under cold running water. Transfer to a large bowl.

Step 2 :Meanwhile, combine vinegar, maple syrup and a large pinch of salt in a bowl. Add cabbage and toss to coat. Set aside for 10 minutes to pickle. Drain.

Step 3 :Combine tahini, lemon juice, oil and 1-2 tbs warm water in a small bowl until smooth.

Step 4 :Divide pasta mixture, pickled cabbage, carrot and tofu among serving bowls. Drizzle over the dressing and sprinkle with pepitas.

RECIPE NOTES

Use buckwheat pasta for a gluten-free version. This recipe is part of our 2019 7-day kickstart meal plan.

VEGAN PANCAKE RECIPE

INGREDIENTS

- 2 cups self-raising flour
- 1/2 cup caster sugar
- 1 1/2 cups unsweetened rice milk
- 2 tsp vanilla bean paste
- 2 tsp baking powder
- 1 tbsp apple cider vinegar
- 2 tbsp coconut oil, melted
- Maple syrup, to serve
- Mixed berries, to serve
- Coconut yoghurt, to serve

METHOD

Step 1 :Place flour and sugar in a large bowl. Stir to combine. Make a well. Place milk and vanilla in a large jug. Add baking powder, then vinegar. Lightly whisk with a fork until frothy. Add to well. Stir until mixture is smooth and just combined. Set aside for 15 minutes (see notes).

Step 2 :Heat a large non-stick frying pan over medium-low heat. Brush pan with coconut oil. Spoon 1/4 cup batter into pan, spreading to form a 12cm round. Repeat to make 2 pancakes. Cook for 3 to 4 minutes or until bubbles appear on surface. Turn and cook for 1 to 2 minutes or until cooked through. Transfer to a plate. Cover loosely with foil to keep warm. Repeat with remaining mixture, brushing pan with oil between batches.

Step 3 :Serve pancakes with maple syrup, mixed berries and yoghurt.

HEALTHY VEGAN TACOS

INGREDIENTS

- 1 tsp paprika
- 1/2 tsp dried chilli flakes
- 1 tsp ground cumin
- 500g butternut pumpkin, peeled, deseeded, cut into 2cm pieces
- 1 large red capsicum, deseeded, cut into 2cm pieces
- 400g can black beans, rinsed, drained
- 2 tsp pure maple syrup
- 2 tbsp fresh lemon juice
- 1/4 small red cabbage, shredded
- 95g (1/3 cup) natural coconut yoghurt
- 3 tsp tahini
- 8 small gluten-free corn tortillas
- 1/2 small avocado, thinly sliced
- Lemon wedges, to serve

METHOD

Step 1 :Preheat oven to 200C/180C fan forced. Line a large baking tray with baking paper. Combine the paprika, chilli flakes and cumin in a small bowl. Place the pumpkin and capsicum on prepared tray. Lightly spray with oil. Sprinkle with the spice mixture. Roast for 30 minutes or until golden and tender, adding the black beans to the tray for the last 5 minutes of cooking. Use a fork to lightly mash the black beans after cooking.

Step 2 :Meanwhile, combine the maple syrup, 1 tbs lemon juice and a large pinch of sea salt flakes in a large bowl. Add the cabbage. Toss to combine. Set aside for 5 minutes to pickle. Drain.

Step 3 :Combine yoghurt, tahini and remaining lemon juice in a small bowl until smooth. Preheat a chargrill pan over high heat (see tip). Cook tortillas 2-3 minutes each side.

Step 4 :Divide pickled cabbage among tortillas. Top with roast vegetables, sliced avocado and a dollop of tahini yoghurt. Season with pepper and serve with lemon wedges.

VEGAN VANILLA SLICE

INGREDIENTS

- 2 sheets frozen puff pastry, partially thawed (see notes)
- 1 vanilla bean, split
- 1 litre Soy Milky
- 1 cup caster sugar
- 1 1/3 cups cornflour
- 100g Nuttelex original spread
- 1/4 tsp ground turmeric
- 1/3 cup icing sugar mixture

METHOD

Step 1 :Preheat oven to 200C/180C fan-forced. Line 2 large baking trays with baking paper. Place 1 pastry sheet on each tray. Bake pastry for 15 minutes or until golden, puffed and cooked through. Allow to cool for 5 minutes, then gently flatten pastry using your hand. Cool completely.

Step 2 :Meanwhile, grease a 6cm-deep, 22cm square cake pan. Line base and sides with baking paper, extending paper 2cm above edges of pan.

Step 3 :Using a sharp knife, scrape seeds from vanilla bean. Place Soy Milky, vanilla bean and seeds in a saucepan over medium heat. Cook, stirring, for 10 minutes or until almost simmering (don't boil). Set aside for 10 minutes for flavours to infuse. Strain. Discard bean.

Step 4 :Place 1 sheet of pastry in prepared pan, trimming sheet if necessary. Place caster sugar and cornflour in a large, heavy-based saucepan. Gradually add Milky mixture, stirring constantly with a wooden spoon, until smooth and combined. Place over medium heat. Cook, stirring constantly, for 8 to 10 minutes or until mixture bubbles and thickens. Stir in Nuttelex and turmeric. Working quickly, remove from heat. Spoon hot 'custard' mixture over pastry. Top with second pastry sheet, trimming if necessary. Set aside to cool for 30 minutes. Refrigerate for 4 hours or until cold and firm.

Step 5 :Remove vanilla slice from pan. Place on a board. Dust with icing sugar. Cut into squares. Serve.

LEMON AND LIME VEGAN TARTS

INGREDIENTS

- 1 1/2 cups (225g) cashews
- 1 cup (160g) whole almonds
- 1/4 cup (35g) pistachios
- 1/2 cup (40g) shredded coconut
- Pinch of salt
- 12 fresh dates, pitted, chopped
- 270ml can coconut cream
- 1 lemon, rind finely grated, juiced
- 1 lime, rind finely grated, juiced
- 1/3 cup (80ml) maple syrup
- Lemon & lime slices, to serve
- Lemon & lime zest, to serve
- Mint leaves, to serve

METHOD

Step 1 :Place the cashews in a large bowl. Pour over enough boiling water to cover. Set aside for 4 hours to soak.

Step 2 :Lightly grease eight 8cm (base measurement) fluted tart tins with removable bases. Place the tins on a baking tray.

Step 3 :Place almonds, pistachios, shredded coconut and salt in a food processor. Process until finely chopped. Add dates. Process until very finely chopped and mixture holds together when pinched. Spoon mixture evenly among prepared tins. Use the back of the spoon to press mixture evenly over base and side of each tin. Place in the freezer to set.

Step 4 :Drain cashews. Place in a blender with the coconut cream, lemon rind, lemon juice, lime rind, lime juice and ¼ cup (60ml) of the maple syrup. Blend until mixture is very smooth and creamy. Pour mixture evenly among tart cases in the tins. Gently tap on bench to smooth surfaces. Freeze for 2 hours or until firm.

Step 5 :Transfer the tarts to serving plates. Top with lemon and lime slices, lemon and lime zest and mint. Drizzle with remaining maple syrup. Serve frozen or at room temperature.

VEGAN CHOCOLATE

INGREDIENTS

- 250g Flora Plant Original spread
- 3 cups (660g) caster sugar
- 1/3 cup (35g) dairy-free cocoa powder
- 1 tsp bicarbonate of soda
- 3 cups (405g) gluten-free self-rising flour
- 1 cup (300g) Coles apple sauce
- 1/2 cup (50g) psyllium husk
- Mixed berries, to serve

CHOCOLATE FROSTING

- 150g Flora Plant Original spread
- 2 cups (300g) gluten-free icing sugar mixture
- 1/2 cup (50g) dairy-free cocoa powder
- 1 tbs vanilla bean paste
- 1 1/2 tbs dairy-free milk (such as oat milk)

- EQUIPMENT
- 2 x 20cm (base measurement) round cake pans

METHOD

Step 1 :Combine the Flora Plant Original, sugar, cocoa powder, bicarbonate of soda and 2 cups (500ml) water in a large saucepan over medium heat. Cook, stirring, for 5 mins or until the sugar dissolves. Increase heat to high and bring to the boil. Set aside for 20 mins to cool.

Step 2 :Preheat oven to 180°C. Grease two 20cm (base measurement) round cake pans and line the bases and sides with baking paper.

Step 3 :Whisk flour, apple sauce and psyllium husk into the chocolate mixture in the saucepan. Divide the mixture among the prepared pans. Bake for 1 hour or until a skewer inserted in the centres comes out clean. Set aside in pans for 5 mins to cool slightly before turning onto a wire rack to cool completely.

Step 4 :To make chocolate frosting, use an electric mixer to beat Flora Plant Original in a bowl until creamy. Add icing sugar and cocoa powder, in 3 batches, beating well after each addition. Beat in the vanilla and milk until smooth.

Step 5 :Place 1 cake on a serving plate. Spread top with 1/2 cup of frosting. Top with remaining cake. Spread top and side of entire cake with remaining frosting. Decorate with berries.

VEGAN MEDITERRANEAN

INGREDIENTS

- 4 x 200g capsicums (2 yellow, 2 red)
- 450g packet microwave brown rice, warmed
- 400g can black beans, rinsed, drained
- 60g (1/3 cup) semi-dried tomato strips in oil, undrained
- 1 small zucchini, coarsely grated
- 1/3 cup chopped fresh continental parsley leaves and stems
- 1 tablespoon finely grated lemon rind
- 2 green shallots, finely chopped
- 2 garlic cloves, crushed
- 60ml (1/4 cup) Massel Vegetable Liquid Stock
- 60ml (1/4 cup) avocado oil
- Bought vegan basil pesto, to serve

METHOD

Step 1 :Preheat oven to 200°C/180°C fan forced. Use a small sharp knife to cut the tops off the capsicums, reserving the lids. Use a teaspoon to scoop out the seeds and remove the membranes. Arrange the capsicum shells, cut-side up, in a small roasting pan.

Step 2 :Combine the rice, beans, tomato strips, zucchini, parsley, lemon rind, shallot, garlic and stock in a large bowl. Season.

Step 3 :Divide the rice mixture among the capsicum shells, pressing down lightly as you fill. Place reserved lids on top. Drizzle over the oil. Cover with foil.

Step 4 :Bake for 25 minutes. Remove the foil and bake for a further 15 minutes or until the capsicum shells are just tender. Top filling with pesto and replace lids to serve.

CRISPY VEGAN NOODLE SALAD

INGREDIENTS

- 100g snow peas
- 2 teaspoons vegetable oil
- 200g Japanese teriyaki tofu
- 150g (2 cups) finely shredded red cabbage
- 1 yellow capsicum, deseeded, cut into thin strips
- 2 small carrots, cut into thin strips
- 1 Lebanese cucumber, thinly sliced
- 125g cherry tomatoes, halved
- 40g (1/2 cup) Chang's Original Fried Noodles
- 15g (1/4 cup) fried shallots
- DRESSING
- 80ml (1/3 cup) vegan mayonnaise
- 1 1/2 tablespoons fresh lime juice
- 1 teaspoon sesame oil
- 1/2 teaspoon Sriracha chilli sauce, or to taste

METHOD

Step 1 :Prepare a bowl of iced water. Place the snow peas in a heatproof bowl. Pour boiling water over the snow peas. Set aside for 30 seconds to blanch. Drain and plunge immediately into the iced water. Drain and pat dry with paper towel. Trim the ends and cut lengthways into thin strips.

Step 2 :Heat the oil in a large frying pan over medium heat. Cook the tofu for 2 minutes each side or until golden brown. Transfer to a plate. Set aside to cool slightly. Slice.

Step 3 :To make the dressing, whisk all the ingredients in a small bowl.

Step 4 :Combine the cabbage, capsicum, carrot, cucumber, tomato and most of the noodles on a large platter or shallow bowl. Top with the tofu and drizzle with half the dressing. Sprinkle with the shallots and remaining noodles, and serve with the remaining dressing on the side.

VEGAN CHICKPEA SATAY CURRY

INGREDIENTS

- oil 1 tbsp peanut
- 1 brown onion, cut into thin wedges
- 2 garlic cloves, crushed
- 1 tsp crushed red chilli (or sambal olek)
- 90g (1/3 cup) Sanitarium™ Natural Smooth Peanut Butter
- 160ml (2/3 cup) coconut milk
- 2 tbsp light soy sauce
- 700g pumpkin, peeled, deseeded, cut into 2cm pieces
- 160ml (2/3 cup) water
- 200g green beans, trimmed, halved
- 400g can Coles Chickpeas, drained, rinsed
- 1 tbsp fresh lime juice
- 1/4 cup fresh coriander leaves
- Steamed brown rice, to serve

METHOD

Step 1 :Heat the oil in a large, deep frying pan or wok over medium heat. Add the onion and cook, stirring occasionally, for 5 minutes or until soft and lightly golden. Add the garlic and chilli and cook, stirring, for 30 seconds or until aromatic.

Step 2 :Reduce the heat to low and add the peanut butter, coconut milk and soy sauce. Stir until evenly combined. Add the pumpkin and 160ml (2/3 cup) water. Cover and bring to a simmer. Cook, stirring occasionally, for 6 minutes or until the pumpkin is just tender.

Step 3 :Add the beans and chickpeas to the pan and cook for a further 2 minutes or until beans are tender-crisp. Stir in lime juice and top with coriander leaves. Serve with brown rice.

VEGAN STUFFED ROAST PUMPKIN

INGREDIENTS

- 1.8kg whole butternut pumpkin
- 2 red onions
- 1 tbsp extra virgin olive oil
- 3 garlic cloves, thinly sliced
- 1 tsp smoked paprika
- 2 small red capsicums deseeded, cut into 1cm-thick strips
- 2 small yellow capsicums, deseeded, cut into 1cm-thick strips
- 2 tbsp red wine vinegar
- 2 tsp pure maple syrup
- 400g can brown lentils, rinsed, drained
- 150g baby spinach
- 2 tbsp pine nuts
- 2 bunches asparagus, trimmed
- Baby rocket, to serve
- Balsamic vinegar, to serve

METHOD

Step 1 :Preheat oven to 190C/170C fan forced. Line a large baking tray with baking paper. Cut pumpkin in half lengthways. Scoop out seeds. Place the pumpkin, cut-side up, on prepared tray. Lightly spray with oil. Season. Roast for 1 hour 10 minutes or until tender. Cut 1 onion into wedges. Thinly slice the remaining onion. Set aside pumpkin to cool then scoop out flesh from each pumpkin half, leaving a 3cm-thick shell. Reserve flesh.

Step 2 :Meanwhile, heat oil in a large frying pan over medium heat. Cook sliced onion, stirring, for 3 minutes or until softened. Add the garlic and paprika. Cook, stirring, for 1 minute. Add capsicum and cook, stirring occasionally, for 10 minutes or until just tender. Stir in vinegar and maple syrup. Cook, stirring occasionally, for 10-15 minutes or until caramelised.

Step 3 :Add lentils and reserved pumpkin to onion mixture. Season. Stir. Set aside to cool slightly.

Step 4 :Blanch spinach in boiling water. Drain. Refresh under cold running water. Squeeze out excess liquid then coarsely chop. Stir through the lentil mixture with pine nuts.

Step 5 :Divide lentil mixture between pumpkin shells. Carefully join halves and use kitchen string to tie at 2cm intervals. Return pumpkin to tray. Add onion wedges. Roast for 20 minutes or until just tender, adding asparagus halfway through cooking. Set aside for 5 minutes. Remove string. Cut into 6 thick slices. Arrange on serving plates with asparagus, onion and rocket. Drizzle over balsamic.

VEGAN 'ICED VOVO' FROZEN CHEESECAKE

INGREDIENTS

- 400g raw cashew nuts
- 2 tsp finely grated lemon rind
- 1 tsp vanilla bean paste
- 270ml can light coconut milk
- 2 tbsp pure maple syrup
- 10g freeze-dried raspberries
- 300g fresh raspberries
- 20g (1/4 cup) desiccated coconut, plus extra, to serve
- BASE
- 30g natural almonds
- 25g (1/4 cup) rolled oats
- 45g (1/2 cup) desiccated coconut
- 80g fresh dates, pitted
- 1 tbsp coconut oil
- 1 tsp vanilla bean paste

METHOD

Step 1 : Grease a 20cm square cake pan and line the base and sides with baking paper.

Step 2 : Place 250g cashews in a bowl and the remaining 150g cashews in a separate bowl. Cover both with boiling water. Set aside for at least 2 hours to soak.

Step 3 : Meanwhile, to make the base, place the almonds and oats in a food processor and process until finely chopped. Add the coconut and process to combine. Add the dates, coconut oil and vanilla. Process until well combined. Use the back of a spoon to press mixture over base of prepared pan. Smooth surface. Place in the fridge to chill.

Step 4 : Drain the 250g cashews and place in a blender with the lemon rind, vanilla, 200ml coconut milk and 1 tbs maple syrup. Blend, occasionally scraping down the side of the blender, for 2-3 minutes or until thick and very smooth. Spread evenly over the base. Cover and place in the freezer until required.

Step 5 : Drain the remaining cashews and place in a clean blender with the freeze-dried raspberries, 175g fresh raspberries and remaining coconut milk and maple syrup. Blend, occasionally scraping down the side of the blender, for 2-3 minutes or until thick and very smooth. Carefully spread over the vanilla cashew layer. Sprinkle with the coconut.

Step 6 : Use a fork to crush the remaining fresh raspberries and arrange in 4 lines over the cheesecake, well spaced apart. Cover and place in the freezer for 3-4 hours or until firm.

Step 7 : Sprinkle the cheesecake with extra coconut. Set aside for 10 minutes before cutting into squares. Store in the freezer until ready to serve.

SATAY NOODLE STIR-FRY VEGAN

INGREDIENTS

- 100g dried edamame bean fettuccine pasta
- 1 tsp sesame oil
- 350g broccoli, cut into florets
- 2 large carrots, peeled, cut into matchsticks
- 1 red capsicum, deseeded, thinly sliced
- 4 green shallots, thinly sliced, plus extra, thinly sliced, to serve
- 2 garlic cloves, crushed
- 100g podded frozen edamame
- 200g satay-marinated tofu, cut into long strips
- 2 tbsp salt-reduced soy sauce

METHOD

Step 1 :Place the pasta in a large heatproof bowl. Cover with boiling water. Set aside for 5 minutes or until softened. Drain.

Step 2 :Heat the oil in a large wok over high heat. Stir-fry the broccoli, carrot, capsicum, shallot and garlic for 2 minutes or until almost tender. Add edamame and tofu. Stir-fry for 1 minute. Add the pasta and soy sauce. Stir-fry for 1-2 minutes or until hot. Serve topped with extra shallot.

VEGAN 'MEATBALL' SKEWERS WITH GREEN HUMMUS

INGREDIENTS

- 1 small red onion, thinly sliced
- 1 tbsp fresh lemon juice
- 16 vegan 'meatballs'
- 1 Lebanese (slender) eggplant, cut into 1cm-thick pieces
- 1 zucchini, cut into 1cm-thick pieces
- 8 button mushrooms
- 8 cherry tomatoes
- 1 yellow capsicum, deseeded, cut into 2cm pieces
- 4 large wholemeal flatbread
- 200g finely shredded red cabbage
- Fresh mint leaves, to serve
- GREEN HUMMUS
- 400g can chickpeas, rinsed, drained
- 80g baby spinach
- 2 garlic cloves, coarsely chopped
- 2 tbsp fresh lemon juice
- 1 tbsp tahini

METHOD

Step 1 :Vegan meatballs stacked with fresh veg make scrumptious skewers, particularly when devoured in a wrap with hummus and slaw.

Step 2 :Preheat a barbecue grill or large chargrill pan on medium-high. Combine the onion and lemon juice in a bowl. Set aside to pickle.

Step 3 :Meanwhile, thread the 'meatballs', eggplant, zucchini, mushroom, tomato and capsicum onto 8 metal or presoaked bamboo skewers. Brush generously with olive oil.

Step 4 :Grill the flatbread for 1-2 minutes each side then wrap in a clean tea towel to keep warm and soft. Place the skewers onto the grill and cook, turning occasionally, for 6-8 minutes or until vegetables are soft and lightly charred.

Step 5 :Spread the green hummus onto the flatbread. Top each piece with the cabbage and 2 skewers. Sprinkle with the pickled onion and mint to serve.

VEGAN AND GLUTEN-FREE CHRISTMAS CAKE

INGREDIENTS

- 185g Nuttelex original 2 tbsp flaxseed meal
- dairy-free spread
- 1 cup almond meal
- 1 cup gluten-free buckwheat flour
- 1/3 cup Brazil nuts
- 1/3 cup pecans
- 1/3 cup halved macadamia nuts
- 1/4 cup pistachio kernels
- 1 1/2 tbsp brandy
- CRANBERRY AND FIG FRUIT MINCE
- 1 cup sultanas
- 1 cup dried figs, finely chopped
- 1/2 cup dried pitted prunes, finely chopped
- 1/2 cup currants
- 1/2 cup dried cranberries
- 2 tsp finely grated orange rind
- 1/2 cup tawny fortified wine
- 1 1/2 tsp mixed spice

- 1 cinnamon stick
- 1 star anise
- 2/3 cup dark brown sugar

METHOD

Step 1 : Place all ingredients in an airtight container. Stir to combine. Secure lid. Store in a cool, dark place for at least 1 week, stirring every 2 days, to allow flavours to develop (see notes).

Step 2 : Preheat oven to 150C/130C fan-forced. Grease a 7cm-deep, 19cm (base) square cake pan (see notes). Line base and sides of pan with 1 layer of brown paper and 2 layers of baking paper, extending paper 5cm above edges of pan.

Step 3 : Place fruit mince in a large bowl. Discard star anise and cinnamon. Place flaxseed and 3/4 cup water in a medium bowl. Stir well. Stand for 2 minutes or until mixture thickens. Meanwhile, add dairy-free spread to fruit mince. Stir until well combined. Add flaxseed mixture. Stir until well combined. Add almond meal and flour. Stir until well combined.

Step 4 : Spread mixture into prepared pan. Level top with a spatula. Using the picture as a guide, decorate cake with nuts.

Step 5 : Bake for 2 hours or until a skewer inserted in centre comes out clean. Brush hot cake with brandy. Stand for 5 minutes. Fold paper over top of cake and turn, in pan and upside-down, onto a tray lined with baking paper. Cover with a clean tea towel. Cool cake in pan overnight. Serve (see notes).

VEGAN JAPANESE STUFFED SWEET POTATOES

INGREDIENTS

- 4 small (about 200g each) scrubbed sweet potatoes
- 1 1/2 tablespoons mirin
- 1 tablespoon miso paste
- 2 teaspoons salt-reduced soy sauce
- 1 teaspoon sesame oil
- 250g firm tofu, cut into 1cm cubes
- 145g (1 cup) podded frozen edamame
- 1/4 small red cabbage, shredded
- 4 green shallots, thinly sliced
- 2 teaspoons finely grated fresh ginger
- 2 teaspoons toasted sesame seeds

METHOD

Step 1 :Preheat the oven to 200C/180C fan forced. Use a fork or skewer to prick sweet potatoes all over. Place on a baking tray and roast, turning once, for 50 minutes or until tender when pierced with a skewer.

Step 2 :Meanwhile, combine mirin, miso, soy sauce and oil in a small bowl. Lightly spray a non-stick wok with olive oil and heat over high heat. Stir-fry tofu, in 2 batches, for 2-3 minutes or until golden. Transfer to a plate. Reduce heat to medium-high and spray wok with a little more oil. Add edamame, cabbage, shallot and ginger. Stir-fry for 2 minutes or until just tender. Return tofu to the wok with half the miso mixture and stir-fry for 1 minute or until heated through.

Step 3 :Cut a slit in each potato. Use a fork to lightly mash flesh. Spoon filling into each potato. Top with remaining miso mixture and sesame.

VEGAN SOBA NOODLE SALAD WITH SPICY PEANUT DRESSING

INGREDIENTS

- 180g soba noodles
- 1/2 cup podded frozen edamame
- 1 large carrot, peeled, halved
- 1/2 bunch radishes, trimmed
- 1 Lebanese cucumber, halved, deseeded
- 1 avocado, finely chopped
- Chopped roasted peanuts, to serve
- PEANUT DRESSING
- 70g (1/4 cup) natural crunchy peanut butter
- 1 lime, juiced
- 1 tbs mirin
- 1 tbs tamari
- 2 tsp sriracha chilli sauce
- 2 tsp maple syrup

METHOD

Step 1 :Cook the soba noodles in a saucepan of boiling water following packet directions, adding the edamame in the last minute of cooking. Drain. Refresh under cold running water. Transfer to a large serving bowl.

Step 2 :Meanwhile, to make the peanut dressing, combine all ingredients in a bowl. Whisk until smooth.

Step 3 :Use a food processor fitted with the grater attachment to grate the carrot, radish and cucumber then add to bowl with noodles. Add the dressing and half the avocado. Toss well to combine. Top with remaining avocado and sprinkle with peanuts to serve.

CREAMY VEGAN SUN-DRIED TOMATO AND BROCCOLINI GNOCCHI

INGREDIENTS

- 1 garlic clove
- 1 bunch broccolini
- 500g pkt fresh mini or regular-sized gnocchi
- 150g (1 cup) frozen peas
- 100g sun-dried tomato strips, 1 tbs oil reserved from jar
- 1 tbs plain flour
- 375ml (1 1/2 cups) So Good Almond Original milk
- Fresh basil leaves, to serve

METHOD

Step 1 : Put the kettle on.

Step 2 : While the kettle boils, crush the garlic and cut the broccolini stalks in half lengthways. Heat a deep frying pan over medium-high heat.

Step 3 :Pour the boiling water into a large saucepan over high heat. (Don't fill too high or it will take too long to boil again.) Add the gnocchi and cook until gnocchi rise to the surface, adding the peas and broccolini in the last minute of cooking. Drain.

Step 4 :Once the frying pan is hot, pour in the reserved sun-dried tomato oil. Add the garlic and cook, stirring, for 30 seconds. Add the flour. Cook, stirring, for 30 seconds. Remove from heat and gradually whisk in the almond milk until well combined. Return to a medium heat and cook, stirring constantly, until the mixture boils. Simmer for 3 minutes or until the sauce thickens slightly. Season.

Step 5 :Add the gnocchi mixture and tomato strips to the sauce and stir to combine. Divide among serving bowls, season and top with basil.

CREAMY VEGAN TOMATO SOUP WITH SPINACH AND RICOTTA RAVIOLI

INGREDIENTS

- 1 tbsp extra virgin olive oil
- 1 brown onion, chopped
- 2 garlic cloves, chopped
- 800g can whole peeled tomatoes
- 1 large potato, peeled, diced
- 2 cups Massel Vegetable Liquid Stock
- 1 tsp dried oregano
- 1 cup almond milk
- 300g packet vegan spinach and ricotta ravioli
- 150g baby spinach
- Baby spinach, plus extra to serve
- Extra virgin olive oil, to serve
- Fresh basil leaves, to serve

METHOD

Step 1 :Heat oil in a large saucepan over medium-high heat. Add onion and garlic. Season with salt and pepper. Cook, stirring occasionally, for 6 minutes or until softened. Add tomato, potato, stock and oregano. Bring to the boil. Cover. Reduce heat to medium. Simmer for 20 minutes.

Step 2 :Remove from heat. Add almond milk. Using a stick blender, carefully blend mixture until smooth. Keep warm.

Step 3 :Cook pasta following packet directions. Drain. Add spinach to soup. Stir until starting to wilt. Divide soup among serving bowls. Add pasta. Season with pepper. Drizzle with a little extra oil. Serve topped with basil and extra spinach.

ICE-CUBE TRAY VEGAN CHEESECAKE BITES

INGREDIENTS

- cashews 110g (2/3 cup) raw
- 80ml (1/3 cup) cup coconut cream
- 60ml (1/4 cup) maple syrup
- 1 tablespoon fresh lemon juice
- 1 teaspoon vanilla extract
- 2 tablespoons coconut oil, melted, cooled
- 12 raspberries, chopped
- 6 chocolate ripple biscuits, crushed

METHOD

Step 1 :Place the cashews in a glass or ceramic bowl and cover with cold water. Cover with plastic wrap and set aside for 8 hours or overnight to soak.

Step 2 :Cut 12 small strips of baking paper and use to 'line' twelve 40ml (2-tablespoon) ice cube moulds, extending up the side of each.

Step 3 :Drain the cashews and transfer to a blender. Add the coconut cream, maple syrup, lemon juice, vanilla extract and 1 tablespoon of the coconut oil. Blend until smooth.

Step 4 :Divide the raspberries among each ice cube mould and pour the cashew mixture over. Place in the freezer for 20 minutes or until just firm.

Step 5 :Mix the crushed biscuits and remaining 1 tablespoon of coconut oil together. Spoon evenly over each cheesecake bite and press with the back of a spoon. Freeze for 2 hours or until set. Slide a knife down each side of a cheesecake bite to loosen and then use the baking paper strips to ease the cheesecake bites out of the moulds.

PLANT POWER POTATO SALAD WITH VEGAN DRESSING

INGREDIENTS

- 600g baby Red Royal potatoes, skins on, cut into 2-3cm pieces
- 150g bag chopped kale
- 2 tbsp baby capers, drained on paper towel
- 1-2 cloves garlic, crushed
- 70g (1/4 cup) coconut yoghurt
- 1 tbsp Dijon mustard
- 2-3 tsp apple cider vinegar
- 1-2 celery sticks, thinly sliced
- 200g (1 cup) sauerkraut
- 1 small red onion, thinly sliced
- 85g (1/3 cup) walnuts, toasted, optional
- Pomegranate arils, to serve, optional

METHOD

Step 1 :Preheat oven to 180C/160C fan forced. Line a large baking tray with non-stick baking paper. Cook potatoes in a large saucepan of boiling water for 10-15 minutes or until just tender but still holding shape.

Step 2 :Spread kale and capers over oven tray and spray with oil. Add garlic and toss, rubbing in with your fingertips. Season. Bake for 10-12 minutes or until bright green and crisp.

Step 3 :Whisk yoghurt, mustard and vinegar in a small bowl. Season. Thin with water if needed.

Step 4 :Drain warm potatoes and transfer to a large bowl. Pour over dressing and toss to combine. Divide potatoes between serving bowls. Top with celery, sauerkraut and onion. Scatter over crispy kale and capers. Serve with toasted walnuts and pomegranate arils if desired.

VEGAN TAHINI BISCUITS

INGREDIENTS

- 2 teaspoons lemon juice
- 1/4 teaspoon bicarbonate of soda
- 3/4 cup caster sugar
- 1/3 cup hulled tahini
- 1 teaspoon finely grated lemon rind
- 1/4 cup olive oil
- 1/4 cup Freenut butter (see note)
- 1 cup plain flour
- 1/2 teaspoon baking powder
- 1 teaspoon ground cinnamon
- 1/2 teaspoon ground mixed spice
- 1/4 cup sesame seeds

METHOD

Step 1 :Preheat oven to 180°C/160°C fan-forced. Line 2 baking trays with baking paper.

Step 2 :Combine juice and bicarbonate of soda in a glass bowl (mixture will become foamy). Add sugar, tahini, lemon rind, oil and Freenut butter. Using an electric mixer, beat for 1 minute or until mixture is just combined. Sift flour, baking powder, cinnamon and mixed spice over tahini. Add sesame seeds. Beat on low until just combined.

Step 3 :Roll 2 level teaspoons of mixture into balls. Place on prepared trays, 4cm apart. Flatten slightly with a fork.

Step 4 :Bake for 15 minutes, swapping trays halfway during cooking, or until golden and cooked through. Stand on trays for 5 minutes. Cool on a wire rack. Serve.

VEGAN CHICKPEA SATAY CURRY

INGREDIENTS

- 1 tbsp peanut oil
- 1 brown onion, cut into thin wedges
- 2 garlic cloves, crushed
- 1 tsp crushed red chilli (or sambal olek)
- 90g (1/3 cup) Sanitarium™ Natural Smooth Peanut Butter
- 160ml (2/3 cup) coconut milk
- 2 tbsp light soy sauce
- 700g pumpkin, peeled, deseeded, cut into 2cm pieces
- 160ml (2/3 cup) water
- 200g green beans, trimmed, halved
- 400g can Coles Chickpeas, drained, rinsed
- 1 tbsp fresh lime juice
- 1/4 cup fresh coriander leaves
- Steamed brown rice, to serve

METHOD

Step 1 :Heat the oil in a large, deep frying pan or wok over medium heat. Add the onion and cook, stirring occasionally, for 5 minutes or until soft and lightly golden. Add the garlic and chilli and cook, stirring, for 30 seconds or until aromatic.

Step 2 :Reduce the heat to low and add the peanut butter, coconut milk and soy sauce. Stir until evenly combined. Add the pumpkin and 160ml (2/3 cup) water. Cover and bring to a simmer. Cook, stirring occasionally, for 6 minutes or until the pumpkin is just tender.

Step 3 :Add the beans and chickpeas to the pan and cook for a further 2 minutes or until beans are tender-crisp. Stir in lime juice and top with coriander leaves. Serve with brown rice.

RECIPE NOTES

Use peanut butter with no salt or sugar.

CREAMY VEGAN TOMATO SOUP WITH SPINACH AND RICOTTA RAVIOLI

INGREDIENTS

- 1 tbsp extra virgin olive oil
- 1 brown onion, chopped
- 2 garlic cloves, chopped
- 800g can whole peeled tomatoes
- 1 large potato, peeled, diced
- 2 cups Massel Vegetable Liquid Stock
- 1 tsp dried oregano
- 1 cup almond milk
- 300g packet vegan spinach and ricotta ravioli
- 150g baby spinach
- Baby spinach, plus extra to serve
- Extra virgin olive oil, to serve
- Fresh basil leaves, to serve

METHOD

Step 1 :Heat oil in a large saucepan over medium-high heat. Add onion and garlic. Season with salt and pepper. Cook, stirring occasionally, for 6 minutes or until softened. Add tomato, potato, stock and oregano. Bring to the boil. Cover. Reduce heat to medium. Simmer for 20 minutes.

Step 2 :Remove from heat. Add almond milk. Using a stick blender, carefully blend mixture until smooth. Keep warm.

Step 3 :Cook pasta following packet directions. Drain. Add spinach to soup. Stir until starting to wilt. Divide soup among serving bowls. Add pasta. Season with pepper. Drizzle with a little extra oil. Serve topped with basil and extra spinach.

CREAMY VEGAN SUN-DRIED TOMATO AND BROCCOLINI GNOCCHI

INGREDIENTS

- 1 garlic clove
- 1 bunch broccolini
- 500g pkt fresh mini or regular-sized gnocchi
- 150g (1 cup) frozen peas
- 100g sun-dried tomato strips, 1 tbs oil reserved from jar
- 1 tbs plain flour
- 375ml (1 1/2 cups) So Good Almond Original milk
- Fresh basil leaves, to serve

METHOD

Step 1 : Put the kettle on.

Step 2 : While the kettle boils, crush the garlic and cut the broccolini stalks in half lengthways. Heat a deep frying pan over medium-high heat.

Step 3 :Pour the boiling water into a large saucepan over high heat. (Don't fill too high or it will take too long to boil again.) Add the gnocchi and cook until gnocchi rise to the surface, adding the peas and broccolini in the last minute of cooking. Drain.

Step 4 :Once the frying pan is hot, pour in the reserved sun-dried tomato oil. Add the garlic and cook, stirring, for 30 seconds. Add the flour. Cook, stirring, for 30 seconds. Remove from heat and gradually whisk in the almond milk until well combined. Return to a medium heat and cook, stirring constantly, until the mixture boils. Simmer for 3 minutes or until the sauce thickens slightly. Season.

Step 5 :Add the gnocchi mixture and tomato strips to the sauce and stir to combine. Divide among serving bowls, season and top with basil.

VEGAN STUFFED ROAST PUMPKIN

INGREDIENTS

- 1.8kg whole butternut pumpkin
- 2 red onions
- 1 tbsp extra virgin olive oil
- 3 garlic cloves, thinly sliced
- 1 tsp smoked paprika
- 2 small red capsicums deseeded, cut into 1cm-thick strips
- 2 small yellow capsicums, deseeded, cut into 1cm-thick strips
- 2 tbsp red wine vinegar
- 2 tsp pure maple syrup
- 400g can brown lentils, rinsed, drained
- 150g baby spinach
- 2 tbsp pine nuts
- 2 bunches asparagus, trimmed
- Baby rocket, to serve
- Balsamic vinegar, to serve

METHOD

Step 1 :Preheat oven to 190C/170C fan forced. Line a large baking tray with baking paper. Cut pumpkin in half lengthways. Scoop out seeds. Place the pumpkin, cut-side up, on prepared tray. Lightly spray with oil. Season. Roast for 1 hour 10 minutes or until tender. Cut 1 onion into wedges. Thinly slice the remaining onion. Set aside pumpkin to cool then scoop out flesh from each pumpkin half, leaving a 3cm-thick shell. Reserve flesh.

Step 2 :Meanwhile, heat oil in a large frying pan over medium heat. Cook sliced onion, stirring, for 3 minutes or until softened. Add the garlic and paprika. Cook, stirring, for 1 minute. Add capsicum and cook, stirring occasionally, for 10 minutes or until just tender. Stir in vinegar and maple syrup. Cook, stirring occasionally, for 10-15 minutes or until caramelised.

Step 3 :Add lentils and reserved pumpkin to onion mixture. Season. Stir. Set aside to cool slightly.

Step 4 :Blanch spinach in boiling water. Drain. Refresh under cold running water. Squeeze out excess liquid then coarsely chop. Stir through the lentil mixture with pine nuts.

Step 5 :Divide lentil mixture between pumpkin shells. Carefully join halves and use kitchen string to tie at 2cm intervals. Return pumpkin to tray. Add onion wedges. Roast for 20 minutes or until just tender, adding asparagus halfway through cooking. Set aside for 5 minutes. Remove string. Cut into 6 thick slices. Arrange on serving plates with asparagus, onion and rocket. Drizzle over balsamic.

COOKIES RECIPES

CUTE CRITTER COOKIES

INGREDIENTS

- 12 digestive biscuits
- 1 cup (160g) icing sugar mixture
- 50g pkt Nestlé Smarties
- Chocolate writing icing
- Red liquid food colouring
- 20g pkt Coles Funny Face Icing Figurines
- Brown Mars M&M's Minis

METHOD

Step 1: Place the digestive biscuits on a serving plate.

Step 2: Place the icing sugar in a bowl. Stir in enough cold water to make a smooth paste.

Step 3: To make butterflies and caterpillars, spread two-thirds of the icing over 8 of the biscuits. Decorate with Smarties and writing icing. Set aside to set.

Step 4: To make ladybirds, tint the remaining icing red. Spread red icing over the remaining biscuits. Decorate with Funny Face Icing Figurine eyes, writing icing and M&M's. Set aside to set.

ALMOND AND CHERRY COOKIES

INGREDIENTS

- 160g butter, softened
- 1/2 cup (110g) Coles Caster Sugar
- 2 Coles Australian Free Range Eggs
- 1 tsp almond essence
- 1/4 tsp pink liquid food colouring
- 2 cups (300g) plain flour
- 1 cup (120g) almond meal
- 200g pkt red glacé cherries, coarsely chopped
- 1/2 cup (70g) pistachios, coarsely chopped
- 1/2 cup (40g) desiccated coconut

METHOD

Step 1: Line 2 baking trays with baking paper. Use an electric mixer to beat the butter, sugar, eggs, almond essence and food colouring in a large bowl until well combined. Stir in the flour and almond meal. Add the cherry and pistachio and stir until well combined.

Step 2: Turn the dough onto a lightly floured surface and gently knead until smooth. Divide into 2 even portions. Roll each portion into a 22cm log. Place the coconut on a plate. Roll the logs in coconut to coat. Cover with plastic wrap. Place in the fridge for 30 mins to chill.

Step 3: Preheat oven to 160°C. Cut the logs into 1cm-thick slices. Place the slices on the trays, about 3cm apart. Bake for 20 mins or until golden and firm. Transfer the cookies to a wire rack to cool completely.

RECIPE NOTES

Allow for cooling and 30 minutes chilling time.

SLICE IT RIGHT - For perfectly round slices, chill the log for 30 mins before slicing – too soft and the log won't retain its shape as you cut.

FREEZE THE DOUGH - Freeze in an airtight container for up to 3 months. Slice and bake from frozen for 23-25 mins or until golden and firm.

BANANA COOKIES

INGREDIENTS

COOKIE DOUGH BASE

- 125g salted butter, softened
- 1/2 cup brown sugar
- 1/4 cup caster sugar
- 1 egg
- 1 cup traditional rolled oats
- 1/2 cup self-raising flour
- 1/2 cup wholemeal self-raising flour

BANANA COOKIES

- 1 ripe banana, mashed
- 1/2 cup roughly chopped banana chips
- 100g dark chocolate, melted

METHOD

Step 1: Using an electric mixer, beat butter and sugars until pale and creamy. Add egg. Beat well to combine. Add oats and flours. Stir with a wooden spoon to combine.

Step 2: Preheat oven to 190°C/170°C fan-forced. Line 2 baking trays with baking paper. Add banana and chips to dough. Stir to combine. Refrigerate for 45 minutes to firm slightly.

Step 3: Roll 2 level tablespoons of mixture into 16 balls. Place onto prepared trays, allowing room for spreading. Using the palm of your hand, slightly flatten to form a 5.5cm round. Bake for 12 to 14 minutes, swapping trays after 10 minutes, or until light golden. Stand cookies on trays for 5 minutes. Transfer to a wire rack to cool.

Step 4: Place cookies on a sheet of baking paper. Spoon chocolate into a snap-lock bag. Snip off one corner. Drizzle chocolate over cookies. Stand until chocolate sets. Serve.

TRASH COOKIES

INGREDIENTS

- 1 1/2 cups plain flour
- 1/2 tsp cream of tartar
- 1/2 tsp bicarbonate of soda
- 3/4 cup caster sugar
- 125g butter, melted, cooled
- 2 tsp vanilla extract
- 1 egg, lightly beaten
- 1/2 cup jelly beans
- 1 1/3 cups mini pretzels
- 1 cup mixed M&M's
- 12.5g sachet Wizz Fizz sherbert

METHOD

Step 1: Preheat oven to 180C/160C fan-forced. Grease 4 large baking trays. Line with baking paper.

Step 2: Sift flour, cream of tartar and bicarbonate of soda into a large bowl. Stir in sugar. Add butter, vanilla and egg. Mix well to combine. Roll level tablespoons of mixture into balls. Flatten each ball into a disc and place on prepared trays, 5cm apart. Top with jelly beans, pretzels and M&M's, pressing to secure.

Step 3: Bake cookies, 2 trays at a time, for 12 to 15 minutes or until just turning golden around the edges. Cool on trays for 5 minutes. Transfer to a wire rack to cool completely. Dust with sherbert. Serve.

RECIPE NOTES

You will need to pile the toppings liberally onto the biscuits, as the biscuits spread a lot during cooking.

MILO THUMBPRINT COOKIES

INGREDIENTS

- 125g butter, softened
- 1 tsp vanilla extract
- 1/2 cup firmly packed brown sugar
- 1 egg
- 1/2 cup Milo
- 1/2 cup almond meal
- 1 1/4 cups plain flour
- 1/4 cup strawberry jam

METHOD

Step 1: Preheat oven to 180C/160C fan-forced. Line 2 large baking trays with baking paper.

Step 2: Using an electric mixer, beat butter, vanilla and sugar in a bowl until light and fluffy. Add egg, beating well to combine. Using a wooden spoon, stir in Milo, almond meal and flour until combined.

Step 3: Using damp hands, roll 2 level tablespoons of mixture into balls. Place balls onto prepared baking trays 6cm apart to allow room for spreading. Flatten slightly. Using your thumb or the back of a spoon, make a 3cm-wide indentation in the centre of each cookie. Fill each hole with 1/2 teaspoon jam.

Step 4: Bake for 15 to 20 minutes, swapping trays after 10 minutes, or until light golden. Using remaining jam, top up holes with another 1/2 teaspoon jam. Cool on trays. Serve.

APRICOT AND PISTACHIO COOKIES

INGREDIENTS

COOKIE DOUGH BASE

- 125g salted butter, softened
- 1/2 cup brown sugar
- 1/4 cup caster sugar
- 1 egg
- 1 cup traditional rolled oats
- 1/2 cup self-raising flour
- 1/2 cup wholemeal self-raising flour

APRICOT AND PISTACHIO COOKIES

- 2 tbsp sunflower kernels
- 1 tbsp white chia seeds
- 1/2 tsp ground cinnamon
- 2 tbsp finely chopped dried apricots

- 2 tbsp finely chopped pistachio kernels

METHOD

Step 1: Using an electric mixer, beat butter and sugars until pale and creamy. Add egg. Beat well to combine. Add oats and flours. Stir with a wooden spoon to combine.

Step 2: Preheat oven to 190°C/170°C fan-forced. Line 2 baking trays with baking paper. Add sunflower kernels, chia seeds and cinnamon to dough. Stir to combine.

Step 3: Roll 2 level tablespoons of mixture into 16 balls. Place onto prepared trays, allowing room for spreading. Using the palm of your hand, slightly flatten to form a 5.5cm round. Top with apricots and pistachios. Bake for 15 minutes, swapping trays after 10 minutes, or until light golden. Stand cookies on trays for 5 minutes. Transfer to a wire rack to cool. Serve.

CHOCOLATE AND COCONUT COOKIES

INGREDIENTS

COOKIE DOUGH BASE

- 125g salted butter, softened
- 1/2 cup brown sugar
- 1/4 cup caster sugar
- 1 egg
- 1 cup traditional rolled oats
- 1/2 cup self-raising flour
- 1/2 cup wholemeal self-raising flour

CHOLOATE AND COCONUT COOKIES

- 1 quantity cookie dough base
- 3/4 cup coconut flakes, roughly chopped
- 2 tbsp dark chocolate chips

METHOD

Step 1: Using an electric mixer, beat butter and sugars until pale and creamy. Add egg. Beat well to combine. Add oats and flours. Stir with a wooden spoon to combine.

Step 2: Preheat oven to 190°C/170°C fan-forced. Line 2 baking trays with baking paper. Add ½ cup coconut to dough. Stir to combine.

Step 3: Roll 2 level tablespoons of mixture into 16 balls. Place onto prepared trays, allowing room for spreading. Using the palm of your hand, slightly flatten to form a 5.5cm round. Top with chocolate chips and remaining coconut. Bake for 15 minutes, swapping trays after 10 minutes, or until light golden. Stand cookies on trays for 5 minutes. Transfer to a wire rack to cool. Serve.

CHOCOLATE CHILLI COOKIES

INGREDIENTS

COOKIE DOUGH BASE

- 125g salted butter, softened
- 1/2 cup brown sugar
- 1/4 cup caster sugar
- 1 egg
- 1 cup traditional rolled oats
- 1/2 cup self-rising flour
- 1/2 cup wholemeal self-raising flour

CHOCOLATE CHILLI COOKIES

- 100g dark chocolate, melted
- 1 tsp ground cinnamon
- 1/2 tsp vanilla bean paste
- Pinch dried red chilli flakes

METHOD

Step 1: Using an electric mixer, beat butter and sugars until pale and creamy. Add egg. Beat well to combine. Add oats and flours. Stir with a wooden spoon to combine.

Step 2: Preheat oven to 190°C/170°C fan-forced. Line 2 baking trays with baking paper. Add melted chocolate, cinnamon and vanilla to basic dough. Stir to combine.

Step 3: Roll 2 level tablespoons of mixture into 16 balls. Place onto prepared trays, allowing room for spreading. Using the palm of your hand, slightly flatten to form a 5.5cm round. Sprinkle with chilli flakes. Bake for 15 minutes, swapping trays after 10 minutes, or until light golden. Stand cookies on trays for 5 minutes before transferring to a wire rack to cool. Serve.

EASY KITKAT COOKIES

INGREDIENTS

- 2 x 170g blocks Nestlé KitKat
- 225g unsalted butter, softened
- 75g (1/3 cup) caster sugar
- 180ml (3/4 cup) Nestlé Sweetened Condensed Milk
- 300g (2 cups) plain flour
- 1 tsp baking powder
- 200g pkt Nestlé Bakers' Choice Milk Choc Bits
- 2 tbsp Nestlé Bakers' Choice Cocoa Powder

METHOD

Step 1: Preheat oven to 190C/170C fan-forced. Grease and line three large baking trays.

Step 2: Open the blocks of KitKat and chop 10 fingers into thirds (so you have 30 small pieces in total) and set aside. Finely chop remaining fingers.

Step 3: Using an electric mixer, beat butter and sugar until pale and creamy. Beat in sweetened condensed milk. Sift the flour and baking powder together and stir into butter mixture until combined. Stir in milk chic bits and finely chopped KitKat.

Step 4: Spoon 1/3 of the cookie mixture into a bowl and stir in the cocoa powder until combined. Return cocoa mixture to the remaining cookie mixture and mix gently to swirl both mixtures together.

Step 5: Roll level tablespoons of mixture into balls and place, 5cm apart, on prepared trays. Bake for 15 minutes or until golden. Top each hot cookie with a piece of KitKat and press in gently. Set aside to cool. Serve.

CHOCKY ROCK COOKIES

INGREDIENTS

- 125g butter
- 1/2 cup (110g) caster sugar
- 1 Coles Australian Free Range Egg, lightly whisked
- 1 cup (150g) plain flour
- 1/2 tsp baking powder
- 1/2 cup (80g) sultanas
- 2/3 cup (130g) dark chocolate chips
- 1/2 cup (45g) rolled oats
- 2 cups (80g) cornflakes

METHOD

Step 1: Preheat oven to 180°C. Line 2 large baking trays with baking paper. Use an electric mixer to beat the butter and sugar in a large bowl until pale and creamy. Add the egg and beat until well combined. Add the flour and baking powder and stir to combine.

Step 2: Add the sultanas, chocolate chips, oats and half the cornflakes to the flour mixture. Stir to combine.

Step 3: Place the remaining cornflakes in a medium bowl and use a wooden spoon to lightly crush.

Step 4: Roll 1-tbs portions of the sultana mixture into balls, then dip in the crushed cornflakes to lightly coat. Place on the lined trays. Flatten slightly.

Step 5: Bake, swapping the trays halfway through cooking, for 15 mins or until light golden. Transfer to a wire rack to cool completely.

CRANBERRY LEMON COOKIES

INGREDIENTS

COOKIE DOUGH BASE

- 125g salted butter, softened
- 1/2 cup brown sugar
- 1/4 cup caster sugar
- 1 egg
- 1 cup traditional rolled oats
- 1/2 cup self-raising flour
- 1/2 cup wholemeal self-raising flour

CRANBERRY LEMON COOKIES

- 1 tbsp finely grated lemon rind
- 1 tbsp lemon juice
- 1/2 cup finely chopped dried cranberries

METHOD

Step 1: Using an electric mixer, beat butter and sugars until pale and creamy. Add egg. Beat well to combine. Add oats and flours. Stir with a wooden spoon to combine.

Step 2: Preheat oven to 190°C/170°C fan-forced. Line 2 baking trays with baking paper. Add lemon rind and juice and half the cranberries to dough. Stir to combine.

Step 3: Roll 2 level tablespoons of mixture into 16 balls. Place onto prepared trays, allowing room for spreading. Using the palm of your hand, slightly flatten to form a 5.5cm round. Top with remaining cranberries. Bake for 15 minutes, swapping trays after 10 minutes, or until light golden. Stand cookies on trays for 5 minutes. Transfer to a wire rack to cool. Serve.

TAHINI AND HONEY COOKIES

INGREDIENTS

COOKIE DOUGH BASE

- 125g salted butter, softened
- 1/2 cup brown sugar
- 1/4 cup caster sugar
- 1 egg
- 1 cup traditional rolled oats
- 1/2 cup self-raising flour
- 1/2 cup wholemeal self-raising flour

TAHINI AND HONEY COOKIES

- 2 tbsp tahini
- 1 tbsp honey
- 2 tbsp pepitas
- 2 tsp sesame seeds

METHOD

Step 1: Using an electric mixer, beat butter and sugars until pale and creamy. Add egg. Beat well to combine. Add oats and flours. Stir with a wooden spoon to combine.

Step 2: Preheat oven to 190°C/170°C fan-forced. Line 2 baking trays with baking paper. Add tahini and honey to dough. Stir to combine.

Step 3: Roll 2 level tablespoons of mixture into 16 balls. Place onto prepared trays, allowing room for spreading. Using the palm of your hand, slightly flatten to form a 5.5cm round. Sprinkle with pepitas and sesame seeds. Bake for 15 minutes, swapping trays after 10 minutes, or until light golden. Stand cookies on trays for 5 minutes. Transfer to a wire rack to cool. Serve.

CHOC DIPPED FORTUNE COOKIES

INGREDIENTS

- 100 pkt fortune cookies
- 100g white chocolate, melted
- Pink liquid food colouring
- Blue liquid food colouring
- Coles Funfetti Sprinkles, to decorate
- Coles Star Sprinkles, to decorate

METHOD

Step 1: Line a large baking tray with baking paper. Unwrap the cookies and place on the lined tray.

Step 2: Divide the chocolate into 3 bowls. Use food colouring to tint 2 of the chocolate portions pale pink and blue.

Step 3: Working quickly, dip 1 cookie halfway into melted chocolate. Return to tray. Repeat with remaining cookies and chocolate.

Step 4: Sprinkle some of the cookies with the funfetti sprinkles and star sprinkles. Set. Place any remaining chocolate into separate sealable bags. Cut off 1 small corner. Drizzle over some of the cookies. Set.

VEGAN CHOC-CHIP COOKIES

INGREDIENTS

- 110g Nuttelex vegan olive oil spread
- 150g (3/4 cup) coconut sugar
- 1 teaspoon pure vanilla extract
- 235g (1 1/2 cups) wholemeal spelt flour
- 1 teaspoon ground cinnamon
- 60ml (1/4 cup) unsweetened almond milk
- 80g vegan milk chocolate, chopped

METHOD

Step 1: Preheat oven 180C/160C fan forced. Line a large baking tray with baking paper. Use electric beaters to beat the spread, sugar and vanilla in a bowl until pale and creamy.

Step 2: Sift the flour and cinnamon into the spread mixture. Add the milk and chocolate. Stir until well combined and a soft sticky dough forms.

Step 3: Use slightly wetted hands to roll tablespoonfuls of the mixture into balls. Place on the prepared tray, about 5cm apart. Flatten well with a fork. Bake for 12 minutes or until golden. Transfer to a wire rack to cool completely.

PEANUT BUTTER SANDWICH COOKIES

INGREDIENTS

- 3/4 cup Lakanto Monkfruit Golden Sweetener
- 1/2 cup butter unsalted, melted
- 3/4 cup peanut butter
- 1 whole egg
- 1 1/2 cups coconut flour
- 1 tsp vanilla essence
- 1/4 cup peanut butter (to fill)

METHOD

Step 1: Combine the sweetener and melted butter, peanut butter and lightly beaten egg. Mix well.

Step 2 Gradually add sifted flour and remaining ingredients, mixing thoroughly.

Step 3: Place teaspoons of mixture onto a greased tray, flattening with a fork.

Step 4: Bake for about 12-15 minutes at 160C.

Step 5: Allow to cool before sandwiching with peanut butter. Serve.

SUPER-EASY JELLY COOKIES

INGREDIENTS

- 250g butter, softened
- 1/4 cup caster sugar
- 1 egg
- 2 1/2 cups plain flour
- 85g packet lime-flavoured jelly crystals
- 85g packet raspberry-flavoured jelly crystals
- 85g packet orange-flavoured jelly crystals
- 1/4 cup boiling water

METHOD

Step 1: Using an electric mixer, beat butter and sugar until pale and creamy. Add egg. Beat until combined. Sift flour over butter mixture. Beat until combined. Divide dough into 3 equal portions.

Step 2: Place jelly crystals in 3 separate bowls. Working with one flavour at a time, add 1 tablespoon boiling water. Whisk to combine (crystals will not dissolve completely). Add 1 portion of dough. Stir with a wooden spoon until well combined. Place on a sheet of plastic wrap. Using plastic wrap to avoid dough sticking to your fingers, shape into an 18cm-long log. Repeat with remaining jelly crystals, boiling water and dough to make 3 logs. Freeze for 30 minutes.

Step 3: Preheat oven to 180C/160C fan-forced. Line 3 large baking trays with baking paper.

Step 4: Remove 1 dough log from freezer. Slice log into 1cm-thick rounds. Roll each round into a ball. Place balls, 3cm apart, on one of the prepared trays. Press down slightly with palm of hand. Repeat with remaining dough logs. Bake for 12 minutes or until light golden. Cool on trays for 5 minutes. Transfer to a wire rack to cool completely. Serve.

CRUNCHY NUTTY CORNFLAKE COOKIES

INGREDIENTS

- 125g butter, softened
- 1/3 cup caster sugar
- 1/3 cup firmly packed brown sugar
- 1 teaspoon ground ginger
- 3/4 cup wholemeal self-raising flour
- 1/2 cup self-raising flour
- 1/4 cup milk
- 2 cups cornflakes
- 22 pecans

METHOD

Step 1: Preheat oven to 180C/160C fan-forced. Line 2 large baking trays with baking paper.

Step 2: Using an electric mixer, beat butter, sugars and ginger in a bowl until light and fluffy. Add flours. Beat on low speed until just combined. Add milk. Beat until dough comes together. Using a wooden spoon, stir in cornflakes.

Step 3: Using 1 tablespoon of mixture at a time, roll into balls. Place balls 5cm apart on prepared trays to allow room for spreading. Flatten slightly. Top each with 1 pecan. Bake for 12 to 14 minutes, swapping trays after 8 minutes, or until light golden. Stand for 5 minutes on trays. Transfer to a wire rack to cool. Serve.

BAILEY'S CHOCOLATE CHIP COOKIES

INGREDIENTS

- 125g butter, at room temperature, chopped
- 100g (1/2 cup, firmly packed) brown sugar
- 70g (1/3 cup) caster sugar
- 60ml (1/4 cup) Baileys Irish Cream liqueur
- 1 egg
- 200g (1 1/3 cups) plain flour
- 1 teaspoon bicarbonate of soda
- 1/2 teaspoon table salt
- 290g pkt dark chocolate melts, coarsely chopped

METHOD

Step 1: Preheat oven to 180C/160C fan forced. Line 3 large baking trays with baking paper.

Step 2: Use electric beaters to beat the butter, sugars and liqueur in a small bowl until pale and creamy. Add the egg. Beat until well combined. Transfer the mixture to a large bowl. Sift in the flour, bicarb and salt. Stir until just combined. Add the chocolate. Stir until just combined. Place in the fridge for 1 hour to rest.

Step 3: Use slightly damp hands to roll 1 1/2 tablespoonfuls of the mixture into balls. Place the balls, 6cm apart, on the prepared trays. Use the heel of your hand to slightly flatten the balls.

Step 4: Bake for 12-14 minutes or until light golden. Set aside on trays for 5 minutes to cool slightly before transferring to a wire rack to cool completely. Serve.

SANTA PULL-APART COOKIES

INGREDIENTS

- 125g butter, softened
- 1/2 cup (110g) caster sugar
- 1 Coles Australian Free Range Egg
- 1 1/2 cups (225g) plain flour
- 1 tsp vanilla bean paste
- 1 tsp finely grated orange rind
- 1 tsp almond extract
- Pink liquid food colouring, to tint
- 2 brown sugar coated chocolates
- Red liquid food colouring, to tint

ROYAL ICING

- 2 Coles Australian Free Range Egg whites*
- 2 tsp lemon juice
- 3 cups (480g) pure icing sugar, sifted

- Egg white, extra
- Lemon juice, extra

METHOD

Step 1: Use an electric mixer to beat the butter, sugar and egg in a large bowl until just combined. Add flour, vanilla, orange rind and almond extract. Beat until the mixture just comes together.

Step 2: Turn dough onto a lightly floured surface. Gently knead until smooth. Divide into 2 portions and shape into discs. Cover with plastic wrap and place in the fridge for 30 mins to chill.

Step 3: Preheat oven to 180°C. Roll out the dough on a lightly floured surface until 3mm thick. Cut a 14cm-wide moustache shape, a 4cm x 14cm rectangle, a 14cm x 6.5cm triangle, two 4.5cm discs, two 6.5cm squares and twenty 4cm stars from the dough, rerolling excess. Place shapes on lined baking trays. Cool on the trays.

Step 4: Meanwhile, to make the royal icing, whisk the egg whites and lemon juice in a large bowl. Gradually add the icing sugar, stirring after each addition until smooth, adding more icing sugar if necessary to make a thick paste. Divide into 3 portions.

Step 5: To make the face, tint 1 portion of icing pink with liquid food colouring. Place a little pink icing in a piping bag fitted with a 1mm plain nozzle. Pipe around edges of the squares and 1 disc. Add a little egg white and lemon juice to remaining pink icing. Spoon over the centre of the shapes and spread to the edges. Attach the M&M's for eyes. Set.

Step 6: To make the hat, tint 1 portion of icing red with liquid food colouring. Place a little red icing in a piping bag fitted with a 1mm plain nozzle. Pipe around edges of the triangle. Add a little extra egg white and lemon juice to remaining red icing. Spoon into centre of the triangle and spread to edges. Set.

Step 7: To make the beard and hat trimmings, place a little of remaining portion of icing in a piping bag fitted with a 1mm plain nozzle. Pipe around edges of remaining biscuits. Add a little extra egg white and lemon juice to remaining white icing. Spoon over the shapes and spread to edges. Set. Pipe white icing over some of the white biscuits to decorate. Set.

ROCKY ROAD CAKE MIX COOKIES

INGREDIENTS

- 440g packet Green's Classic Chocolate Cake mix, Icing Mix included
- 70g (1/3 cup) dark choc bits, plus extra, to decorate
- 55g (1/3 cup) salted peanuts, coarsely chopped, plus extra, coarsely chopped, to decorate
- 25g (1/3 cup) shredded coconut, plus extra, to decorate
- 20g (1/3 cup) mini marshmallows, plus extra, to decorate
- 75g Lurpak Butter, melted, cooled
- 1 egg, lightly whisked
- 60ml (1/4 cup) boiling water

METHOD

Step 1: Preheat oven to 180°C/160°C fan forced. Line 2 baking trays with baking paper.

Step 2: Place the packet cake mix in a large bowl. Add the choc bits, peanuts, coconut and marshmallows. Make a well in the centre. Add the butter and egg. Use a spatula to stir until well combined.

Step 3: Roll heaped tablespoonfuls of the mixture into balls. Place on prepared trays, allowing room for spreading. Flatten slightly then bake for 10 minutes. Set aside on trays for 5 minutes to cool slightly before transferring to wire racks to cool completely.

Step 4: Place the icing mix and boiling water in a bowl. Stir until smooth. Drizzle icing over the biscuits. Working quickly, sprinkle with the extra choc bits, peanuts, coconut and marshmallows. Set aside for 15 minutes or until icing is set then serve.

PEAR AND WHITE CHOC MISO COOKIES

INGREDIENTS

- 180g butter, chilled, chopped
- 1 1/2 tbs white miso paste
- 1 cup (220g) brown sugar
- 1/4 cup (55g) caster sugar
- 1 egg
- 1 egg yolk
- 1 cup (150g) plain flour
- 1 cup (160g) wholemeal plain flour
- 1 cup (90g) rolled oats
- 2 tsp baking powder
- 1 small green pear, cored, finely chopped
- 60g dried pears, finely chopped
- 1/3 cup (65g) white choc bits
- Thinly sliced pear, to serve

METHOD

Step 1: Preheat oven to 170°C. Line 2 baking trays with baking paper. Place the butter in a saucepan over high heat. Cook, stirring occasionally, for 2-3 mins or until dark brown. Transfer to a large heatproof bowl with the miso paste and whisk to combine. Set aside to cool completely.

Step 2: Add the combined sugar to the butter mixture in the bowl. Use an electric mixer to beat until pale and creamy. Add the egg and egg yolk and beat for 1-2 mins or until well combined and a little paler in colour. Add the combined flour, oats and baking powder and stir to combine. Add the chopped pear, dried pear and choc bits. Stir to combine.

Step 3: Roll 1/4-cup portions of the mixture into balls and flatten slightly. Top each with 1 pear slice. Place on lined trays, about 5cm apart.

Step 4: Bake, swapping the trays halfway through cooking, for 20-25 mins or until golden brown. Set aside on the trays for 10 mins to cool slightly before transferring to a wire rack to cool completely. Store the cookies in an airtight container at room temperature for up to 3 days.

RECIPE NOTES

Allow for cooling time.

Seasonal swap: This recipe also works well with apple. Simply swap the fresh and dried pear for fresh and dried apple.

CHOCOLATE AND CANDY CANE CRUSH COOKIES

INGREDIENTS

- 250g butter, softened
- 3/4 cup (165g) Coles Caster Sugar
- 3/4 cup (165g) brown sugar
- 1 tsp peppermint essence
- 1 Coles Australian Free Range Egg
- 2 cups (300g) plain flour
- 1/4 cup (25g) cocoa powder
- 1 tsp bicarbonate of soda
- 250g pkt dark choc chips
- 375g pkt white chocolate melts
- 3 peppermint candy canes, crushed

METHOD

Step 1: Preheat oven to 180°C. Line 2 baking trays with baking paper.

Use an electric mixer to beat the butter, caster sugar, brown sugar, peppermint essence and egg in a bowl until light and fluffy.

Step 2: Add flour, cocoa powder and bicarbonate of soda, in 2 batches, stirring after each addition. Stir in choc chips. Roll tablespoonfuls of the dough into balls. (To freeze, see tip in notes.)

Step 3: Place half the balls on lined trays, 5cm apart. Bake for 12 mins or until just firm. Set aside on trays to cool. Repeat with the remaining cookie dough balls.

Step 4: Place white chocolate in a medium heatproof bowl over a saucepan of simmering water (make sure the bowl doesn't touch the water). Stir until the chocolate melts and is smooth.

Step 5: Line a baking tray with baking paper. Dip one-half of each cookie in the chocolate and transfer to the lined baking tray. Sprinkle with the crushed candy canes. Set the cookies aside for 20 mins or until set.

CRUNCHY CHOC-CHIP MICROWAVE COOKIES

INGREDIENTS

- 125g butter, chopped
- 1 teaspoon vanilla extract
- 1 egg, lightly beaten
- 1 1/2 cups plain flour
- 1/3 cup firmly packed brown sugar
- 1/4 cup caster sugar
- 1/4 teaspoon bicarbonate of soda
- Pinch of sea salt flakes
- 3/4 cup CADBURY Baking Dark Chocolate Melts, halved
- 1/2 cup dark chocolate chips

METHOD

Step 1: Place butter in a microwave-safe bowl. Microwave on HIGH (100%) for 30 seconds or until melted. Set aside for 2 to 3 minutes to cool.

Step 2: Stir in vanilla and egg until combined. Stir in our, sugar, bicarbonate of soda and salt until combined. Add chocolate. Stir to combine.

Step 3: Using 2 level tablespoons at a time, roll mixture into balls. Between the palms of your hands, flatten balls slightly. Line a microwave-safe plate with baking paper. Place about 4 cookies on prepared plate, allowing room for spreading. Microwave on HIGH (100%) for 2 minutes to 2 minutes 30 seconds or until cooked, but soft to touch. Stand for 1 minute. Transfer to a wire rack to cool.

Step 4: Repeat process with remaining cookies in 4 batches. Serve (see note).

RECIPE NOTES

Store cookies in an airtight container for up to 2 days. For a soft cookie, serve on the day of making.

DOUBLE CHOC-CHIP KALE COOKIES

INGREDIENTS

- 50g green curly kale leaves (see note)
- 125g butter, softened
- 3/4 cup firmly packed brown sugar
- 1 tsp vanilla extract
- 1 egg
- 1 1/4 cups plain flour
- 1/4 cup cocoa powder
- Pinch salt
- 1/2 tsp bicarbonate of soda
- 300g dark chocolate, chopped

METHOD

Step 1: Preheat oven to 180C/160C fan-forced. Line 2 large baking trays with baking paper.

Step 2: Place kale in a food processor. Process until very finely chopped.

Step 3: Using an electric mixer, beat butter, sugar and vanilla until pale and creamy. Add egg. Beat to combine.

Step 4: Sift flour, cocoa, salt and bicarbonate of soda over butter mixture. Stir until just combined. Add kale and 2/3 of the chocolate. Using hands, knead dough in the bowl until well combined.

Step 5: Using 1 tablespoon of mixture at a time, roll mixture into balls. Place balls, 5cm apart, on prepared trays. Using the heel of your hand, flatten balls slightly. Press remaining chocolate into tops of rounds.

Step 6: Bake, swapping trays after 8 minutes, for 12 minutes or until just firm. Stand on trays for 5 minutes. Transfer to a wire rack to cool completely. Serve.

RECIPE NOTES

50g green curly kale is the leaves of approximately 3 stalks with stems removed and discarded.

MUESLI COOKIES

INGREDIENTS

- 3 cups homemade toasted muesli
- 1/2 cup (75g) plain flour
- 100g butter, melted, cooled
- 1/3 cup honey
- 1 egg, lightly beaten

METHOD

Step 1: Preheat oven to 170°C. Line two baking trays with baking paper. Combine muesli and flour in a bowl. Whisk butter, honey and egg together.

Step 2: Add butter mixture to oats and mix well. Set aside for 15 minutes. Roll spoonfuls of mixture into balls and place on trays, 3cm apart. Flatten.

Step 3: Bake for 10 mins. Swap trays halfway through. Cool for 10 mins transfer to a wire rack. Repeat with remaining mixture.

SNOWFLAKE COOKIES

INGREDIENTS

- 250g butter, at room temperature
- 210g (1 1/3 cups) icing sugar mixture
- 1 tsp vanilla bean paste
- 2 eggs
- 525g (3 1/2 cups) plain flour
- 2 egg whites, lightly whisked
- 110g (1/2 cup) white sugar

EQUIPMENT

Thin ribbon or string, for hanging

METHOD

Step 1: Preheat oven to 170°C. Line 2 baking trays with non-stick baking paper. Use an electric beater to beat the butter and icing sugar in a large bowl until pale and creamy. Add the vanilla paste and beat until well combined. Add the eggs, 1 at a time, beating well after each addition.

Step 2: Sift the flour over the butter mixture and use a round-bladed knife in a cutting motion to mix until the mixture starts to come together. Bring the dough together in the bowl and divide into 2 equal portions.

Step 3: Roll out 1 portion of dough on a sheet of non-stick baking paper until 7mm thick. Use 6cm-diameter and 9.5cm-diameter snowflake-shaped pastry cutters to cut snowflakes from the dough. Transfer to the lined trays. Place in the fridge for 15 minutes or until slightly firm.

Step 4: Lightly brush the biscuits with egg white and sprinkle with half the white sugar. Use a skewer to make a hole in the top of each biscuit.

Step 5: Bake in oven for 8 minutes or until the biscuits are golden underneath. Set aside on the trays for 5 minutes to cool before transferring to a wire rack to cool completely. Repeat with remaining dough, egg white and white sugar.

Step 6: Thread a piece of ribbon or string through the hole in the top of 1 biscuit and knot the ends. Repeat with the remaining biscuits.

RECIPE NOTES

Cut as many biscuits as possible from the first rolling of dough. The dough becomes tougher the more it's handled, so biscuits from subsequent rollings will have a tougher texture.

CHOC-CHIP COOKIE MASH-UP

INGREDIENTS

- 250g butter, softened
- 1 cup firmly packed brown sugar
- 1 cup caster sugar
- 2 eggs
- 2 teaspoons vanilla extract
- 2 2/3 cups plain flour
- 1 teaspoon bicarbonate of soda
- 1/2 teaspoon salt
- 2/3 cup dark chocolate chips
- 2 tablespoons cocoa powder
- 2/3 cup white chocolate chips

METHOD

Step 1: Preheat oven to 180C/160C fan-forced. Line 2 large baking trays with baking paper.

Step 2: Using an electric mixer, beat butter and sugars until thick and pale. Add eggs and vanilla. Beat until combined. Sift over 2 1/2 cups flour, bicarbonate of soda and salt. Stir to combine.

Step 3: Transfer half the mixture to a separate bowl. Add remaining flour and dark chocolate chips to 1 portion. Stir until combined. Add cocoa powder and white chocolate chips to remaining portion. Stir until combined. Refrigerate both portions for 30 minutes or until mixtures firm slightly.

Step 4: Using 1 level tablespoon of dough at a time, roll mixtures into balls and place on 2 large plates. Using 1 vanilla dough ball and 1 chocolate dough ball, press and shape balls together to form a large ball (do not roll together as flavours will merge). Repeat with remaining dough balls.

PEANUT AND CHOC CHIP COOKIE CAKE

INGREDIENTS

- 125g butter
- 1/2 cup (140g) crunchy peanut butter
- 1/2 cup (110g) caster sugar
- 1/2 cup (110g) brown sugar
- 1 Coles Australian Free Range Egg
- 1 tsp vanilla bean paste
- 1 1/2 cups (225g) plain flour
- 1 tsp baking powder
- 1/2 cup (95g) dark choc chips
- 1/2 cup (95g) milk choc chips
- 1/2 cup (95g) white choc chips
- 1/4 cup (35g) salted roasted peanuts
- Chocolate and vanilla ice cream, to serve
- Chocolate topping, to serve

METHOD

Step 1: Line a slow cooker with 3 layers of baking paper, allowing the sides to overhang.

Step 2: Use an electric mixer to beat the butter, peanut butter and combined sugar in a bowl until pale and creamy. Add egg and vanilla. Beat to combine.

Step 3: Add the flour and baking powder to the butter mixture. Stir with a wooden spoon until well combined. Stir in half the combined choc chips.

Step 4: Press the mixture evenly over the base of the prepared slow cooker. Sprinkle over the remaining combined choc chips with the peanuts.

Step 5: Cover and cook for 21/2-3 hours on low or until the edge of the cake is cooked through. Uncover and cook for a further 30 mins on low or until the cake is set. Turn slow cooker off. Leave the cake in slow cooker to cool slightly.

Step 6: Use the paper to transfer the cookie cake to a serving board. Cut into slices. Serve warm with the ice cream and chocolate topping.

COOKIES AND CREAM MIXED BERRY CRUMBLES

INGREDIENTS

- 750g Granny Smith apples, peeled, cored, cut into 3cm pieces
- 1 tablespoon caster sugar
- 2 cups frozen mixed berries
- 2 teaspoons vanilla extract
- 1/3 cup raspberry jam
- Double cream, to serve

COOKIE CRUMBLE TOPPING

- 75g butter, chilled, chopped
- 2 tablespoons plain flour
- 1 tablespoon cocoa powder
- 133g packet original Oreo cookies, roughly crushed
- 1/4 cup skinless hazelnuts, finely chopped
- 60g dark chocolate, finely chopped

METHOD

Step 1: Preheat oven to 180C/160C fan-forced.

Step 2: Place apple and sugar in a medium saucepan over medium-high heat. Stir to combine. Cover. Bring to the boil. Reduce heat to low. Simmer for 8 minutes or until apple just starts to soften. Remove from heat. Stir in berries and vanilla.

Step 3: Make Cookie Crumble Topping. Using fingers, rub butter, flour and cocoa together in a bowl. Add cookie, hazelnut and chocolate. Toss to combine.

Step 4: Spoon apple and berry mixture into 4 x 1-cup-capacity baking dishes. Dollop with jam. Sprinkle with crumble. Bake for 25 minutes or until crumble is golden. Stand for 5 minutes. Serve with cream.

DATE AND CHOC-CHIP COOKIE BARS

INGREDIENTS

- 125g butter, softened
- 1/3 cup firmly packed dark brown sugar
- 1/3 cup caster sugar
- 2 teaspoons vanilla extract
- 2 eggs
- 1 cup wholemeal self-raising flour
- 1 cup plain self-raising flour
- 1/2 cup traditional rolled oats
- 2 tablespoons milk
- 10 fresh medjool dates, pitted, chopped
- 1/2 cup dark chocolate chips

METHOD

Step 1: Preheat oven to 180C/160C fan-forced. Grease a 20cm x

30cm lamington pan. Line base and sides with baking paper, extending paper 3cm above long sides.

Step 2: Using an electric mixer, beat butter, sugars and vanilla in a medium bowl until pale and creamy. Add eggs, 1 at a time, beating until just combined. Stir in flours, oats and milk. Stir in dates and 1/3 cup chocolate chips until just combined.

Step 3: Spread mixture into prepared pan. Sprinkle with remaining chocolate chips. Bake for 25 minutes or until firm to touch and golden brown. Cool completely in pan. Cut into bars. Serve.

SPICED GINGER COOKIES

INGREDIENTS

- 170g butter, softened
- 1 1/4 cups firmly packed brown sugar
- 1 egg
- 1/4 cup golden syrup
- 2 cups plain flour
- 2 teaspoons bicarbonate of soda
- 2 teaspoons ground ginger
- 1 teaspoon ground cinnamon
- 1/4 cup raw caster sugar
- 2 tablespoons sliced glace ginger

METHOD

Step 1: Preheat oven to 170C/150C fan-forced. Line 2 large baking trays with baking paper.

Step 2: Using an electric mixer, beat butter and sugar until light and fluffy. Add egg and golden syrup. Beat until combined. Sift flour, bicarbonate of soda, ginger and cinnamon over butter mixture. Using a wooden spoon, stir until combined and a soft dough forms.

Step 3: Place raw caster sugar in a shallow dish. Roll level tablespoons of mixture into balls. Roll balls in sugar to coat evenly. Place on prepared trays, 5cm apart, to allow room for spreading.

Step 4: Using the palm of your hand, flatten slightly. Lightly press 1 piece of ginger into the top of each cookie. Bake for 15 to 18 minutes, swapping trays halfway, or until light golden. Cool on trays for 5 minutes. Transfer to a wire rack to cool completely. Serve.